INSTRUMENTATION
FOR THE
OPERATING ROOM
A Photographic Manual

INSTRUMENTATION
FOR THE
OPERATING ROOM
A Photographic Manual

SHIRLEY M. BROOKS TIGHE
RN, BA, AD in Applied Science in Photography
Consultant for the Operating Room
Portland, Oregon

FIFTH EDITION

with 532 color digital photographs
directed by the author

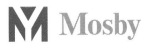 Mosby

St. Louis Baltimore Boston Carlsbad Chicago Minneapolis New York Philadelphia Portland
London Milan Sydney Tokyo Toronto

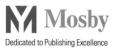

Editor-in-Chief Sally Schrefer
Editor Nancy L. Coon, Loren Wilson
Developmental Editor Nancy L. O'Brien
Project Manager Dana Peick
Senior Production Editor Dottie Martin
Manuscript Editor Carl Masthay
Composition Specialist Dottie Martin
Designer Amy Buxton
Manufacturing Manager Betty Mueller

Lithography/color film by Graphic World
Printing/binding by Von Hoffmann Press

Mosby, Inc.
11830 Westline Industrial Drive
St. Louis, Missouri 63146

Library of Congress Cataloging-in-Publication Data

Brooks Tighe, Shirley M., 1939-
    Instrumentation for the operating room: a photographic manual /
Shirley M. Brooks Tighe. — 5th ed.
        p.   cm.
    Includes bibliographic references and index.
    ISBN 0-323-00350-8
    1. Surgical instruments and apparatus—Atlases. 2. Operating room
nursing.   I. Title.
RD71.B76   1999
617' .9178—DC21   98-53249
                                                          CIP

99 00 01 02 03 / 9 8 7 6 5 4 3 2 1

Contributors

Cynthia C. Spry, RN, MA, MSN, CNOR
International Clinical Consultant
Advanced Sterilization Products
A division of Johnson & Johnson
  Medical, Inc.
Irvine, California
Contributor to "Care and Handling
  of Surgical Instruments"

Susan F. Burdick, RN, CNOR
Operating Room Staff Nurse
Legacy Good Samaritan Hospital
  and Medical Center
Portland, Oregon

Robert A. Burdick, ST
Operating Room Staff Technician
Legacy Good Samaritan Hospital
  and Medical Center
Portland, Oregon

Linda M. Bussey, RN, CNOR
Operating Room Staff Nurse
Legacy Good Samaritan Hospital
  and Medical Center
Portland, Oregon

Gerry J. Casale, RN, CNOR
Perioperative Office Surgical
  Nurse
Tualatin, Oregon

Aloa L. Day, RN
Clinical Resource Nurse
  for Oral, Ear, Nose, Throat
  and Plastic Surgery
Providence St. Vincent Hospital
  and Medical Center
Portland, Oregon

Beverly J. Eagle, RN, CNOR
Coordinator for Eye, Ear, Nose
  and Throat Surgery
Legacy Good Samaritan Hospital
  and Medical Center
Portland, Oregon

Virginia Holbrook, RN
Senior Buyer, Purchasing
Legacy Good Samaritan Hospital
  and Medical Center
Portland, Oregon

Jeanne A. Kauffman, RN, CNOR
Operating Room Staff Nurse
Legacy Good Samaritan Hospital
  and Medical Center
Portland, Oregon

Trudy A.G. Kenyon, RN
Coordinator, Minimal Invasive
  Surgery & Surgical Research
Legacy Emanuel Hospital and
  Medical Center
Portland, Oregon

Frank W. Minnis, ST
Operating Room Staff Technician
Legacy Good Samaritan Hospital
  and Medical Center
Portland, Oregon

Barbara Ann Redman, RN, CNOR
Coordinator for Open Heart and
  Vascular Surgery
Legacy Good Samaritan Hospital
  and Medical Center
Portland, Oregon

Patricia K. Reese, RN
Coordinator for Gynecology,
  Urology and Minimal Invasive
  Surgery
Legacy Good Samaritan Hospital
  and Medical Center
Portland, Oregon

Carol L. Ritzheimer, RN
Evening Coordinator
Legacy Good Samaritan Hospital
  and Medical Center
Portland, Oregon

Cynthia M. Robertson, ST
Operating Room Staff Technician
Legacy Good Samaritan Hospital
  and Medical Center
Portland, Oregon

Mary C. Russell, RN, BSN, CNOR
Urology Speciality Nurse
Portland Veterans' Affairs Medical
  Center
Portland, Oregon

Judith R. Shartel, RN, CNOR
Perioperative Nurse, Cardio-
  Vascular Surgery
Providence St. Vincent Hospital
  and Medical Center
Portland, Oregon

William E. Shellshear
Surgical Supply
  Support/Technician
Legacy Good Samaritan Hospital
  and Medical Center
Portland, Oregon

George W. Stanger, CRCST
Central Sterile Manager
Legacy Good Samaritan Hospital
  and Medical Center
Legacy Emanuel Hospital and
  Medical Center
Portland, Oregon

Pauline A. Svestka, RN
Manager of the Operating Rooms
Legacy Good Samaritan Hospital
  and Medical Center
Portland, Oregon

Lisa M. Van Cleave, CRCST
Central Sterile Specialist
Central Sterile
Legacy Good Samaritan Hospital
  and Medical Center
Portland, Oregon

**Pauline E. Vorderstrasse, RN,
BSN**
Consultant for Operating Rooms
West Linn, Oregon

James G. Wade, RN
Coordinator for Trauma/Neuro
  Surgery and Laser
Legacy Emanuel Hospital and
  Medical Center
Portland, Oregon

James Wiggs, RN, BSN, CNOR
Support Manager
Oregon Health Sciences University
  Hospital
Portland, Oregon

Sue T. Yount, RN, MS, CNOR
Education/Quality Coordinator,
  Surgical Services
Providence Portland Medical
  Center
Portland, Oregon

Jeff Cole
Sales Representative
Ethicon Endo-Surgery
A Johnson-Johnson Company
Portland, Oregon

Bruce Douglas
Digital Photography Specialist
Pro Photo Supply, Inc.
Portland, Oregon

Allan and Marcia Frieze
Case Medical
Ridgefield, New Jersey

A. J. Pasion
President
Zimmer Pasion, Inc.
Beaverton, Oregon

Jack W. Sanders, BA
Assistant Photographer,
Graphic Arts Assistant
Shriners Hospitals for Children
Portland, Oregon

Tammara A. Schuman, RN, MS
Research Associate
Oregon Health Sciences University
Portland, Oregon

Glen E. Tighe
Assistant Photographer
Portland, Oregon

This book is dedicated to the many individuals who shared their expertise to assist with this edition, my contributors. Also to Pauline Svestka, Legacy Good Samaritan Hospital and Medical Center, and Legacy Emanuel Hospital and Medical Center, Portland, Oregon, for providing the photography facilities and the instrumentation.

Preface

This fifth edition is a complete revision of the textbook. It follows the same belief that one must know the basic instrumentation used in surgeries to assist the surgeons in the best possible perioperative care for the patients. It is the concern for the high quality of care we can provide to our patients that helps drive us to always learn and look for new and improved ways of patient care, whether that be through new instrumentation or surgical procedures, improved anesthesia, or simply understanding the real importance of being there and caring for the patients as they undergo what could be a frightening experience.

A digital camera was used for photgraphing the instruments, which allows for improved clarity of the photographs. Therefore the repetition of photographing each instrument is not necessary for the consumer to identify the instruments. This has allowed me to increase the number of procedures by more than 40 while using fewer photographs.

I wish to acknowledge the valuable assistance of the many contributors and friends, for without them this book would not have been possible.

Shirley M. Brooks Tighe

Contents

CARE AND HANDLING OF SURGICAL INSTRUMENTS, 1
Cynthia Spry

Unit Six

NEUROSURGERY

Unit Seven

PERIPHERAL VASCULAR, CARDIOVASCULAR, AND THORACIC SURGERY

Unit Eight

EYE, EAR, NOSE, AND THROAT SURGERY

Unit Nine

ORTHOPEDIC SURGERY

Unit Ten

GENITOURINARY PROCEDURES

Unit Eleven

ORAL, MAXILLARY, AND FACIAL SURGERY

Unit Twelve

PLASTIC SURGERY

Unit Thirteen

PEDIATRIC SURGERY

Care and Handling of Surgical Instruments

Cynthia Spry, RN, MA, MSN, CNOR
International Clinical Consultant
Advanced Sterilization Products

Although evidence exists that stone knives were used to perform surgery as early as 10,000 BC, modern surgical instrumentation began with the introduction of stainless steel in the early 1900s. Approximately 85% of all surgical instrumentation is now made from stainless steel. Although stainless steel continues to comprise the bulk of instrumentation used in surgery today, there have been dramatic changes over the last several decades. One has been the addition of new materials. In addition to stainless steel, Titanium, Vitallium, and various polymers are also used. The introduction of minimally invasive surgery, coupled with the availability of space-age materials, has wrought instrumentation once only dreamed of. Cameras and flexible and rigid endoscopes now make it possible to explore almost every crevice within the human body without having to perform open surgery. Instrument design has focused on enhancing the surgeon's ability to visualize, maneuver, diagnose, and manipulate tissue with increasingly smaller instrumentation. It is possible to repair an aortic aneurysm, perform a coronary artery bypass, operate on a fetus, and so on without a major incision. Advances in instrumentation design have contributed significantly to improved patient outcomes, early discharge, reduced recuperation time, and less physical trauma and pain. The corollary to improved instrument design, however, is higher cost, less inventory of like instrumentation, greater challenge for cleaning and processing, and an even more critical need to properly handle and care for instrumentation. Appropriate care and handling of instrumentation can lower costs that may be incurred for repair or replacement as a result of damage. However, the primary concern should be that the instrument is truly patient ready, that is, safe and appropriately free of microorganisms. Instruments must be in excellent working condition and adequately cleaned and processed in preparation for surgery. Instrumentation that malfunctions or is not appropriately cleaned and sterilized or disinfected can result in extended surgery time, poor technical results, patient infection, patient injury, or even death. Proper care and handling of surgical instrumentation is not a simple rote task; it requires specialized knowledge, competence, judgment, and a commitment to excellent patient care.

EVOLUTION OF SURGERY AND SURGICAL INSTRUMENTATION

Surgery was practiced long before the development of sophisticated surgical instruments. Stone knives, sharpened flints, and animal teeth were the instruments of choice for trephination, circumcision, and blood letting in prehistoric times. In *Corpus Hippocraticum*, Hippocrates (460-377 BC) wrote of the use of iron and steel in instrument making; however, there are no extant examples of surgical instruments before the Early Roman period. Excavations begun in 1771 of the city of Pompeii reveal surgical instruments with amazing resemblance to contemporary instrumentation. Among the instruments found were a foreign-body remover, a speculum, retractors, probes, a periosteal elevator, forceps, spoons, and hooks. Metal analysis indicates three materials: copper, bronze, and iron.

Until the 1790s surgery was not a strict discipline, and surgeons were not afforded equal status with physicians. Instruments were made by blacksmiths, cutlers, and armorers. However, as surgery evolved into a scientific discipline and achieved a measure of status, the specialty of instrument making also emerged. Surgeons employed coppersmiths, steelworkers, silversmiths, wood turners, and other artisans who handcrafted instruments to individual specifications. Instruments often had ornate ivory or carved wooden handles and were cased in velvet.

The introduction of anesthesia in the 1840s and the adoption of Lister's antiseptic technique in the 1880s greatly influenced the making of surgical instruments. The use of anesthesia enabled the surgeon to work more slowly and accurately and to perform longer, more complex procedures. The variety of surgeries performed increased, as did the demand for specialized instruments. The ability to sterilize instruments also had an impact on instrument design. When steam sterilization became a standard process, carved wooden or ivory handles were replaced with all-metal instruments made of silver, brass, and steel. Velvet-lined boxes were replaced with trays that could be lowered into sterilizers.

The development of stainless steel in the 1900s provided a superior material for the manufacture of surgical instruments. Subsequently, instrument making evolved into a highly skilled occupation. Shortly thereafter, craftsmen from Germany, France, and England were brought to the United States to instruct apprentices in their craft. Even today, many of the delicate, high-quality, stainless steel instruments are manufactured in Europe. Other metals like Vitallium and Titanium are used today; however the bulk of surgical instrumentation is made of stainless steel and is manufactured in the United States.

Stainless steel is a compound of varying amounts of carbon, chromium, and iron. Small amounts of nickel, magnesium, and silicone may also be incorporated. Varying the amount of these materials produces a variety of qualities such as flexibility, temper, malleability, and corrosion resistance. There are more than 80 different types of stainless steel. The American Iron and Steel Institute grades steel based on its various qualities. The 400 series stainless steel is most often used for surgical instruments. It resists rust and corrosion, has good tensile strength, and will retain a sharp edge through repeated use. The chromium content in stainless steel provides the stainless quality. Stainless steel is really a misnomer. The degree to which the steel is "stainless" is also determined by the chemical composition of the metal, the heat treatment, and the final rinsing process.

The first step in the manufacture of stainless steel instruments is the conversion of raw steel into sheets that are milled, ground, or lathed into instrument blanks. These blanks are then die-forged into specific pieces and, where appropriate, male and female halves. Excess metal is trimmed away, and the pieces are milled and hand assembled. Jaw serration, ratchet, and shank alignment is achieved, and then the instrument is hand assembled and ground and buffed. It is then heat treated to reach its proper size, weight, spring, temper, and balance. After testing for desired hardness, jaw closure, and ratchet and locking action, a finish is applied.

The final two processes are passivation and polishing. Passivation is the immersion of the instrument in a dilute solution of nitric acid, which removes carbon steel particles and promotes the formation of a coating of chromium oxide on the surface. Chromium oxide is important because it produces corrosion resistance. When carbon particles are removed, tiny pits are left behind. These are removed by polishing, which creates a smooth surface upon which a continuous layer of chromium oxide may form. Passivation and polishing effectively close the instrument's pores and prevent corrosion.

There are three types of finishes: highly polished, satin or dull, and ebony. The highly polished finish reflects light and can cause glare, which may interfere with the surgeon's vision. The satin finish does not reflect light and eliminates glare. The ebony finish is black and also eliminates glare. It is suitable for laser surgery, in which it is critical by being able to prevent the laser from being accidentally reflected and thus diminishing the potential for burn or fire.

Stainless steel instruments may appear to be of uniform quality when they are new. However, there are various grades of quality. Quality ranges from high quality and premium grade to operating room (OR) and floor grade. Some instruments appearing to be stainless steel are of such poor quality that they are sold as single use. In the United States there is no agency that sets standards for instrument quality. Quality is determined by the manufacturer. In addition, an instrument labeled "Germany" may have been forged in Germany but actually assembled in a country where minimum or no quality standards exist. Because instruments represent a substantial portion of a surgical-suite budget, it is important to be knowledgeable about buying and selecting a product with desired quality. Many factors affect quality. Two major factors are a balanced carbon-to-chromium ratio and the process of passivation. A balanced carbon-to-chromium ratio is important for instrument strength and long life. Instruments that are classified as premium have the correct balance. The passivation process is important to create a protective coat as the outer layer of an instrument to prevent corrosion and extend the life. Electropolishing is sometimes substituted for passivation. The result is a less expensive instrument but one that will not last as long. When one is purchasing stainless steel instruments, it is best to deal with a reputable manufacturer who will explain the variation in quality of the products available.

Instruments other than stainless steel present another set of considerations before purchasing. These include the ability to disassemble, clean, and reassemble; life expectancy; and compatibility with existing cleaning, disinfecting, and sterilizing capabilities within the institution.

CARE AND HANDLING OF BASIC SURGICAL INSTRUMENTS—OVERVIEW

A well-made, properly cared for instrument can be expected to last 10 years. The most important considerations in extending the life of an instrument are appropriate use and proper cleaning. Other considerations are disinfection, sterilization, packaging, and storage. Every instrument is designed for a specific purpose. Use for an unintended purpose is a sure method for damaging an instrument. An example of misuse is securing surgical drapes with an instrument designed to grasp tissue.

Proper cleaning of instruments during and after surgery can help prevent stiff joints, malfunction, and deterioration of the stainless steel. During surgery, instruments contaminated with blood or tissue should be properly wiped and rinsed in the distilled water on the sterile field. Thorough rinsing is important to ensure removal of blood and other contaminants from hinges, joints, and crevices. Blood and foreign matter that is allowed to dry and harden may become trapped in jaw serrations, between scissor blades, or in box locks, making final cleaning more difficult. It can cause instruments to become stiff and eventually break. Channels, or lumens, within instruments, such as suction tips, should be irrigated periodically to prevent blood from drying and adhering to the inside of the lumen. Absence of this action can result in blood and other debris remaining in lumens through postoperative cleaning, decontamination, and sterilization processes. A syringe should be present on the sterile field for the purpose of flushing lumens with water throughout the procedure. Instruments should be rinsed in distilled water. Saline should not be used for this purpose. Prolonged exposure to saline solution can result in corrosion and can eventually lead to pitting. Pitting can permit entrapment of debris, interfere with sterilization, and result in the destruction of an instrument.

Instruments should be handled carefully and gently, either individually or in small lots, to avoid possible damage by becoming tangled, dented, and misaligned. During and after surgery they should be placed, not tossed, into the basin. Heavy instruments should be on the bottom with lighter, delicate, and more fragile ones on top. Rigid endoscopes and fiberoptic cables should also be placed on top or separated. Fiberoptic cables should be loosely coiled and never wound tightly. When the procedure is completed, instruments that can be immersed are disassembled, and all box locks are opened. Care should be taken to ensure that they are not tangled or piled high. Instruments are placed in a basin or container with a lid for transport to the decontamination area. Delicate instruments and endoscopes may need to be separated and transported to the decontamination area in specific containers designed to prevent damage. Instruments with cutting edges, pointed tips, and otherwise sharp areas should be placed in such a manner that personnel responsible for cleaning and decontamination are not injured when reaching into the container.

After surgery—cleaning

After surgery, instruments are transported in leakproof containers or trays encased in plastic bags to a designated area for cleaning and decontamination. Instruments should not be transported in basins containing water because the water may spill. The decontamination area may be within the operating room suite or, more often, is located in the central processing department. Instruments that can tolerate immersion and cannot be cleaned immediately should be completely submerged in a warm noncorrosive enzymatic solution and allowed to soak until they can be cleaned. Instruments should be placed horizontally beneath the water, except for laparoscopic-lumened instruments, which should be soaked vertically with the *entire* shaft being submerged. Horizontal soaking of lumens can cause an air bubble to form and prevent the solution from traveling the length of the inner lumen.

All instruments placed on the sterile field for use in a surgical procedure are considered contaminated and should be cleaned whether they were actually used. Blood, saline, or debris can be splashed or inadvertently deposited on any of the instruments; therefore they all require decontamination and processing.

There are several methods for decontamination of instruments; however, all begin with thorough cleaning. Cleaning is followed by a decontamination process, after which the instruments are considered safe to handle but not ready for use. Instrument cleaning can be manual or automatic. Automatic cleaning is preferred where possible. Some specialty instruments and those that cannot tolerate immersion or an automated process require hand washing. Some instruments, because of their design, require manual as well as mechanical cleaning. Examples are laparoscopic instruments and bone reamers. Debris and tissue can easily become trapped in these devices, and mechanical cleaning alone may not be sufficient to remove the debris. Reamers with many crevices may need to be soaked and manually brushed before automatic cleaning. Much will depend on the capability of the automatic cleaners within the decontamination area. Laparoscopic and other lumened instruments should be flushed and brushed. Flushing can be done by attachment of a Luer-Lok syringe, filled with an enzymatic solution, to one of the instrument ports. Brushing must be carried out with a brush long enough to exit the distal end of the shaft. Mechanical washers and ultrasonic irrigators designed for laparoscopic and other lumened devices do an excellent job of cleaning and are preferable.

Several manufacturers have introduced washer-decontaminators to the market. These machines offer a variety of cycles including cool-water rinse, enzyme soaking, washing, ultrasonic cleaning, hot-water rinse, germicide rinse, and drying. After the process, instruments are considered safe to handle. Washer-decontaminators have, to a great extent, replaced manual cleaning or use of a washer-sterilizer.

In a washer-sterilizer the instruments are washed and rinsed and then subjected to a sterilization process. Debris that may not have been removed during the wash phase may become hardened on the instrument during the sterilization phase. For this reason, washer-decontaminators are generally preferred.

At the end of the washer-decontaminator or washer-sterilizer cycle instruments are safe to handle but are not patient ready. They must be inspected, packaged, wrapped, and subjected to a sterilization process to be considered sterile and patient ready.

Detergent should be selected according to the type of debris and tolerance of the instrument. The manufacturer of both the instrument and the mechanical cleaner should be consulted. Detergent pH can be alkaline or acidic. Acidic or heavily alkaline detergent should not be used because either type can destroy the passivation layer and promote corrosion. A low-sudsing detergent with a neutral pH is preferable. High-sudsing detergents may not be completely rinsed and can leave spots and stains on instruments. In areas where water is hard, a water softener should be used to minimize scum and scale formation.

When instruments cannot tolerate immersion, high temperatures, or the pressures of mechanical cleaning units, or if no such unit is available, they must be hand cleaned. Instruments that are hand washed should always be completely immersed and allowed to soak in a detergent germicide. They should be disassembled, and box locks, hinges, and joints should be opened. Serrations, box locks, crevices, and lumens must be brushed to remove embedded particles. Scouring pads, abrasive powders or soaps, or sharp implements should not be used to remove debris because these can destroy the protective coating.

Instruments that are hand washed should always be washed beneath the surface of the water to prevent aerosolation and splashing of debris. Personnel responsible for cleaning must wear personal protective attire to prevent contact with blood or fluid that might contain blood. Protective attire consists of a cap, goggles, mask or face shield, sturdy rubber gloves, and a liquidproof gown or apron. Shoe coverings or liquidproof boots are appropriate where fluid may be expected to pool on the floor.

After manual or mechanical cleaning, instruments should be placed in an ultrasonic cleaner. Ultrasonic cleaning uses high-frequency sound waves that are captured and converted into mechanical vibrations, which rapidly pull debris from every part of the instrument. Ultrasound in combination with hot water and a specially formulated detergent causes microscopic bubbles to form on the instrument's surface. As these bubbles implode (burst inward), they create a vacuum, which draws debris from the instrument. This process is known as "cavitation." Ultrasonic cleaning is especially beneficial for instruments with serrations, box locks, and interstices that are not easily accessible.

After ultrasonic cleaning and before sterilization, the instruments should be rinsed. Ultrasonic cleaning does not kill pathogens; it only removes and deposits them in the ultrasonic bath. Debris removed during ultrasonic cleaning remains suspended in the cleaning solution and can cover instruments as they are removed. Thorough rinsing is necessary to remove this fine debris. Instruments that are stored should be dried to prevent rust formation, corrosion, and spotting.

Ultrasonic cleaning can be accomplished either before or after decontamination in a washer-decontaminator or washer-sterilizer. In either case, the ultrasonic cleaner should be located in the decontamination area as opposed to the clean area where inspection, assembly, packaging, and sterilization occur. The ultrasonic cleaner should be used only after gross debris has been removed from the instruments. The water in the ultrasonic cleaner should be replaced frequently to remove debris that can interfere with the cavitation process. The lid on the ultrasonic cleaner should be closed during operation to prevent spread of aerosols that are created during the process.

Instruments of dissimilar metal can be damaged if cleaned together in the ultrasonic cleaner. In addition, some instruments cannot tolerate the energy waves of the ultrasonic cleaning process, and manufacturers of delicate instruments do not always recommend ultrasonic cleaning. Personnel responsible for processing instruments should check with both the instrument manufacturer and the ultrasonic cleaner manufacturer before employing this process.

As a final step before inspection and packaging for sterilization, instruments should be lubricated with a nonsilicone, water-soluble lubricant.

Specialty instruments

Specialty instruments require exceptional handling. Instruments used in microscopic surgery should be handled separately from those used for general surgery. They are easily tangled and misaligned when heavier general surgical instruments are placed on top of them. Other specialty instruments, such as powered handpieces or telescopes, will be destroyed if subjected to ultrasonic cleaning or a washer-decontaminator or washer-sterilizer cycle and should be meticulously cleaned by hand. Manufacturers' instructions for care and handling should always be followed.

Flexible endoscopes contain long narrow lumens and present a significant challenge to clean. Instructions for cleaning are usually quite detailed and specific. Manufacturers of flexible scopes usually provide in-service education in cleaning and sterilization of these devices. Personnel responsible for cleaning these devices should have thorough knowledge of the process.

Proper cleaning of flexible scopes should begin immediately after use. The lumen should be flushed with an enzymatic solution and the outside wiped to remove gross soil. Debris should not be allowed to dry within the lumen, and the scope should be delivered to the decontamination area as soon as possible after use. The lumen and internal channels should be flushed from the distal end to the proximal end by use of an enzymatic solution. The lumen and channels should be meticulously cleaned with an appropriate-sized brush and then rinsed. The scope may then be cleaned in an automatic scope washer. In absence of an automated system, meticulous manual cleaning according to the manufacturer's recommendation is required.

Spotting, staining, and corrosion

Although stainless steel is highly resistant to spotting, staining, rusting, and pitting, these conditions can occur for many reasons. Understanding the cause of the specific problem usually provides an effective solution.

Minerals in the water may cause light and dark spots. Instruments processed in healthcare facilities where the water supply has a high concentration of minerals may experience spotting. When water droplets condense on the instruments and evaporate slowly, mineral deposits in the water can remain and leave spots. Sodium, calcium, and magnesium minerals are particularly problematic. Use of demineralized water for rinse purposes and pure steam for sterilization may solve the problem. After the sterilization cycle the door to the autoclave should remain closed until all the steam in the chamber is allowed to exhaust. This reduces the amount of condensate remaining on instruments. Vigorous rubbing with a cloth or cleaning with a soft brush may be sufficient to remove mineral-deposit spotting. If spotting remains a problem, the autoclave may need servicing. Leaky or faulty gaskets can be the cause of the problem.

A rust-colored film on instruments may be the result of a high iron content in the water or foreign material within steam pipes. In some instances the installation of a steam filter may help.

Brownish staining can occur when the detergent used for cleaning contains polyphosphates that dissolve copper elements in the sterilizer. The result is that a layer of copper is deposited on the instruments by electrolytic action. If this happens an alternative detergent should be used and the manufacturer's instructions followed.

Black spots are the result of exposure to ammonia, which is found in many cleaning agents. The problem can be resolved by use of an alternative detergent and thorough rinsing. Black stains can also be caused by amine deposits that can be traced to the autoclave steam. Amines are used to clean steam lines. Cleaning of steam lines should be followed with a distilled-water rinse.

Rusting of stainless steel is unlikely, and what often appears to be rust may actually be organic residue in box locks or mineral deposits baked onto the instrument surface. Unless remedied, corrosion may occur.

Actual corrosion is a physical deterioration of the stainless steel. Pitting is a severe form of corrosion in which small pits form on the surface of the instrument. Corrosion and pitting can be caused when instruments are exposed to saline for extended periods of time or when organic debris, such as blood and tissue, are left in difficult-to-clean areas such as box locks, serrations, and ratchets. Detergents that are either too alkaline or too acidic can also cause corrosion and pitting. Detergents with a chlorine base or an acid pH should be avoided. Exposure to phenol (carbolic acid), calcium chloride, ferrous chloride, potassium permanganate, Dakin's solution, and sodium hypochlorite can cause severe pitting. Pitting can also occur when metals of dissimilar composition are cleaned together in an ultrasonic cleaner. To avoid electrolysis, stainless steel instruments should not be mixed with instruments containing aluminum or copper. Improperly cleaned wraps can also create a corrosive environment. The detergent can leak from the wrap during exposure to heat and steam and remain on the instrument.

Measures to avoid instrument corrosion and pitting include soaking instruments after use to prevent debris from drying and hardening, scrubbing hard-to-clean areas, using a neutral pH detergent, thoroughly rinsing with distilled water, and routinely cleaning the sterilizer with water and vinegar to remove impurities.

In summary, the following steps should be taken to prevent spotting, staining, and corrosion:

1. Clean well; remove all soil.
2. Rinse well. When water has a high mineral content, rinse with demineralized water.
3. Select only detergents and disinfecting solutions that are recommended for instruments. Check with instrument and washer-decontaminator or washer-sterilizer manufacturer.
4. When using an ultrasonic cleaner, process instruments with dissimilar metal separately.
5. Dry instruments before wrapping. Ensure adequate drying after exposure to sterilization. Check autoclaves for proper functioning to ensure drying of packs.
6. Have steam lines and boiler periodically inspected to prevent boiler additives from being discharged into the steam.

INSPECTION AND TESTING

Before being packaged, instruments should be inspected for cleanliness, proper function, and absence of defects. An inadequately cleaned, improperly functioning, or damaged instrument is a source of frustration to the surgeon, can cause critical delays in surgery, and can contribute to patient infection or serious injury.

Box locks, serrations, crevices, and other hard to clean areas should be examined for cleanliness. Deposits left on instruments may prevent sterilization from being achieved and may dislodge in the patient.

Box locks should be inspected for minute cracks. Cracks are an indication that breakage is imminent. Jaw movement, jaw alignment, and ratchet function should be checked on all hinged instruments. Joints should work smoothly, and jaws should be in perfect alignment and not overlap. Ratchets should close easily and hold securely. Joint movement can be tested by opening and closing of the instrument several times. The instrument should close and release with ease. Stiff joints can be caused by inadequate cleaning, resulting in minute particles remaining in the joint. Stiffness can also result when water used to clean instruments contains impurities that collect in the joint. Joints that are stiff should be recleaned if necessary and lubricated with a water-soluble lubricant before they are packaged for processing.

One can test jaw alignment by lightly closing the instrument and inspecting the jaws. Any overlap indicates lack of alignment and need for repair. If there are serrations or teeth on the jaws, these should meet and mesh perfectly. One can test this by closing the instrument and holding it up to the light. Light should not be visible through the jaws. Instruments with misaligned jaws can damage tissue and will not effectively occlude bleeders. Misalignment of hemostatic clamps is a common problem most often caused from improper use of the instrument. Hemostatic clamps should not be used as towel clips, needle holders, or pliers or for purposes other than those for which they were designed.

One can test ratchets by clamping the instrument on the first ratchet, holding it at the box lock, and lightly tapping the ratchet portion against a solid object. The instrument should remain closed. Instruments that spring open are faulty and require repair.

The edges of cutting instruments should be inspected for nicks, burrs, and broken tips. Dull, nicked, or dented cutting edges can cause trauma to tissue. Delicate knives, keratomes, needles, and rongeurs can be tested for burrs and rough edges by passing them through kidskin. The sensation of a slight drag is an indication of a burr or a rough edge. Scissors should be tested for cutting ability. Heavy scissors, such as Mayo scissors, should cut easily through four layers of gauze. Metzenbaum and other more delicate scissors should cut easily through two layers of gauze. One of the most frequent complaints regarding instruments is that scissors are not sharp. One solution is to create a schedule for sharpening scissors before edges become dull and problematic. Scissors are most often damaged when used to cut material other than that for which they were designed. One example is the use of Metzenbaum scissors to cut suture material.

Needle holders must hold a needle securely without permitting it to slide or slip during suturing. Needle holders can be tested by grasping the needle in the jaws and locking on the second ratchet. If the needle can be turned easily by hand, it should be tagged for repair. Inappropriate use is a common cause of damage. Needle holders should be selected to match needle size. Using a large needle with a delicate needle holder can spring the jaws of the holder and reduce its holding ability. Needle holders are made to be rejawed. When needle holders no longer hold the needle securely, the jaws need replacement.

Fiberoptic light cords are checked by holding one end up to a light and looking through the other. Broken glass fibers will appear as black dots. The cord should be replaced if more than 20% of the area is affected.

Telescopes should be checked to ensure that the lens is not cloudy or otherwise occluded. Telescopes are checked by holding the scope up to the light and observing the lens image at the distal end. The image should be clear and easily visualized.

Insulated instruments should be checked for breaks in the insulation and for areas where the insulation has separated from the instrument shaft and appears loose. Both are indications that the insulation is not intact. If either defect is observed, the instrument should be removed from service. Loose or nonintact insulation is a serious defect and can result in an unintended burn inside the patient at the point where the insulation is not intact. Insulated instruments are used in laparoscopic surgery where there is a limited field of vision. The site of the burn may not be in the surgeon's field of vision and can go unnoticed. The patient may even be discharged before a complication is noted. In the case of a burn that causes bowel perforation the patient can develop peritonitis, which in turn can lead to additional surgery, extended recovery, and even death from infection.

Microscopic instrumentation should be examined under a microscope to check for burrs or nicks on tips and to check alignment. Some of the teeth on microscopic forceps are very difficult to see with the naked eye, and forceps alignment should be inspected under a microscope.

PREPARATION FOR STERILIZATION

In preparation for sterilization, instruments should be arranged carefully within their sterilization pans or containers. Joints and hinges should be opened, and instruments with multiple parts should be disassembled. Retractors and other heavy instruments should be placed on the bottom, with lighter instruments strung open and placed alongside or on top. Sharp edges should be protected. Delicate, fragile, or lensed instruments should be protected from collision with other instruments in the set. Peel pouches, fingered mats, or plastic holders are examples of items that protect instruments.

Instruments may be processed in wrapped trays or pans or in rigid closed containers that do not require an outer wrap. Rigid container systems provide good instrument protection during sterilization, transport, and storage. They offer the advantage of a sturdy, rigid container that can be stacked without damage to the underlying instrument sets. Because a rigid container offers greater protection than a wrapper, shelf life is potentially increased and the number of times infrequently used sets must be reprocessed is decreased.

Rigid containers may be metal or plastic for steam or ethylene oxide sterilization. Plasma sterilization may have special packaging requirements. Pans and rigid closed container systems should be selected for compatibility with the intended sterilization process.

A towel placed in the bottom of the pan or container helps absorb condensation formed during sterilization and facilitates drying. Instruments that are not completely dry cannot be considered sterile.

Towels or other absorbent material cannot be used in plasma sterilization.

IDENTIFICATION SYSTEMS

Instrument identification systems are used for inventory control, for reordering purposes, and as a deterrent to theft. Color coding and etching are two methods for coding. Color coding may be adapted for a specific instrument set, specialty, department, or surgeon. Most systems use a hard color coating that is permanently fused to the instrument ring handle. For example, a set with green ring handles may indicate that the set belongs within a specific department. Colored tape may be used to manually color code instruments. However, over time the tape may peel or flake or harbor microorganisms.

Another method of instrument identification is etching or engraving the shaft with desired information. Vibrating mechanical engravers that scratch the surface should not be used because they break down the rust-resistant surface of the instrument, potentially allowing corrosion to begin. When a mechanical engraver is used in the area of the box lock, minute fault lines can be created and can result in premature breakage of the lock.

It is important to check with the instrument manufacturer to ensure that the instrument can withstand the desired coding system. Many instrument companies offer engraving upon purchase. If this option is selected, the etching should be performed with an electrochemical etcher, and the etching should be located on the shaft. Electrochemical etching followed by a neutralizing-fluid wash will not harm instruments.

CLASSIFICATION OF INSTRUMENTS

The function of the instruments provides the basis for their classification. Following are general classifications of instruments. Descriptions and examples are included. Names of instruments may vary with the manufacturer, the geographic location within the country, the surgeon's preference, or the healthcare facility in which they are used.

Clamps

Hemostats are used to control the flow of blood. The jaws of a hemostat contain horizontal serrations designed to close the severed edge of a blood vessel with minimal tissue damage. There are several sizes of hemostats. Examples are mosquitos, Criles, Halsteads, and Mayo Peans. The larger hemostats are also used to clamp tissue.

Occluding clamps are used to clamp bowel or vessels that will be reanastomosed. The jaws of occluding clamps used on the bowel contain vertical serrations. Occluding clamps used on blood vessels contain multiple longitudinal rows of finely meshed teeth. Both are designed to prevent leakage while minimizing trauma to the tissue.

Cutting instruments

Knife handles are usually straight handles that hold a variety of knife blades for incisions and dissection. Examples of knife handles are Bard Parker and Beaver. Others, such as Fischer tonsil, Smillie cartilage, and myringotomy knives, incorporate the blade into the structure of the handle.

Although there are many different types of *scissors*, the two basic types are dissection and suture. Dissection scissors are manufactured according to their intended purpose. Small delicate scissors, such as iris or Westcott scissors, are used in ophthalmic, plastic, or microscopic surgery. Metzenbaum scissors are used in intraabdominal and other general surgery. More sturdy scissors, such as Mayo scissors, are appropriate for cutting fascia or suture. Metzenbaum and Mayo scissors are found in most general surgery instrument sets. Curvature, weight, size, and flexibility characteristics vary according to intended use.

Retractors

Retractors are used to hold back the edges of the wound to permit visualization of the operative site. Hand-held retractors consist of a shaft for holding and an end piece for retracting. The end piece may be a hook, a blade, or a rake. Examples of hand-held retractors are skin hook, Senn, Army Navy, Parker, or rake. Self-retaining retractors do not require that someone hold them in place. Some self-retaining retractors consist of two blades that are held apart with a ratchet. Examples are a Weitlaner, Jansen, or Gelpi. Other larger self-retaining retractors consist of a series of blades that attach to bars held in place with a screw or similar device. The bars that hold the blades may be of a kind that is attached to the operating table itself. Examples of larger self-retaining retractors are O'Sullivan O'Connor, Thompson, and Balfour.

Grasping and holding instruments

Forceps, also referred to as pickups, are shaped like tweezers and are used to grasp and hold tissue. The tips of forceps vary according to intended use. The tips may be smooth or serrated or have single or multiple teeth that interlock.

Examples of common clamp-shaped grasping instruments include the Kocher, Allis, and Babcock. The Kocher clamp has a heavy tooth at the jaw tip and is used to grasp and hold tissue without concern for trauma. The Allis clamp has multiple noncrushing teeth and is used to grasp tissue without crushing. The Babcock clamp has a curved, fenestrated tip without teeth. It is useful for grasping structures such as the fallopian tube or ureter.

Needle holders are grasping instruments designed to secure a suture needle in its jaws. Needle holders may be a clamp type with a ratchet handle or may be a spring-action type. Size and jaw surface vary and are selected with regard to the procedure and the size of the needle being used.

A towel clamp is a holding instrument used to secure towels and drapes in place. The tip may be pointed and designed to penetrate, or the tips may be blunt.

A sponge holder is a clamplike instrument with rounded jaws and is used to hold a folded 4-by-4 inch sponge.

Accessory instruments

Suction instruments vary in length, curvature, and lumen diameter and are selected according to the type of surgery and the amount and depth of fluid to be suctioned. Minor, delicate surgery and surgery on small vessels require a small-diameter suction. Two examples of small diameter suctions are Frazier or antrum. Abdominal, deep joint, and other general surgery usually require a Yankauer or Poole suction. Poole suctions are used in areas where fluid is deep. A Yankauer is a curved suction with the suction opening on the tip. A Poole suction is straight with multiple holes along the length of the shaft.

SUMMARY

Surgical instruments are a major financial investment in every surgical facility, and processes should be in place to protect this investment. The life of a surgical instrument is dependent on the way it is used and the care it receives. It is the responsibility of the surgical team and the personnel who process the instruments to handle them carefully, use them for the purpose for which they were designed, and process and maintain them appropriately. The extra time it takes to properly care for instruments is well worth the investment and is always in the patient's best interest.

Bibliography

Baxter Healthcare Corporation, V. Mueller Division (1990). *Atlas of surgical instrument care.* McGraw Park, Ill.: Baxter Healthcare Corp.

DeSchutter C, Ritz S (1996). Processing minimally invasive instrumentation. *Infection Control and Sterilization Technology*, 2, 26-28.

Doderlein G. *Antique medical instruments.* Tuttlingen, Federal Republic of Germany: ERKE AG D-7200. Aesculap.

DesCoteaux JG, Poulin EC, Julien M, Guidoin R (1995). Residual organic debris on processed surgical instruments. *AORN Journal*, 63, 23-25.

Harrison SK, Evans, Jr, WJ, LeBlanc DA, Bush LW (1990, January). Cleaning and decontaminating medical instruments. *Journal of Healthcare Materiel Management*, p.35-41.

Meeker MH, Rothrock J (1995). *Alexander's care of the patient in surgery*, ed. 10, p.132-140. St. Louis: Mosby.

Shrubb FJ (1997). Guidelines for reprocessing and sterilizing rigid endoscopes. *Infection Control and Sterilization Technology*, 3, 26-32.

Skinner G (1984, July 18). The history of surgical instruments. *Nursing Times*, 28-30.

Storz Instrument Co. (1992). *The care and handling of surgical instruments*. St. Louis: Storz (now Bausch & Lomb).

Synthes (March 1986). *Checklist: a guide to care and maintenance of the AO/ASIF instrumentation*. Synthes USA: AO ASIF.

Working Group Instrument Preparation (1986). *Proper maintenance of instruments*. Tuttlingen, Federal Republic of Germany: Aesculap.

Unit One

INSTRUMENT STERILIZING TRAYS

Instrument Sterilizing Trays

1-1 *Top, left to right,* Small sterilizing tray; sterilizing tray lid with filter in place. *Bottom, left to right,* Handle for handling hot trays; 2 seal tags; sterilizing filter.

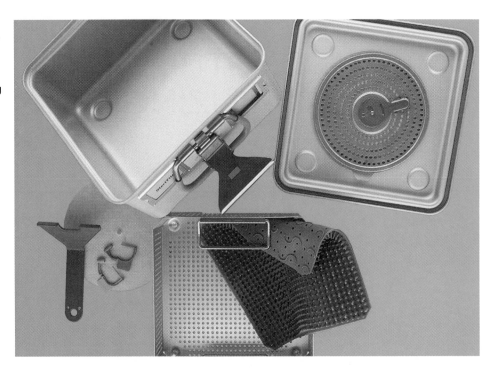

1-2 Instrument holder, marked to assist in instrument count.

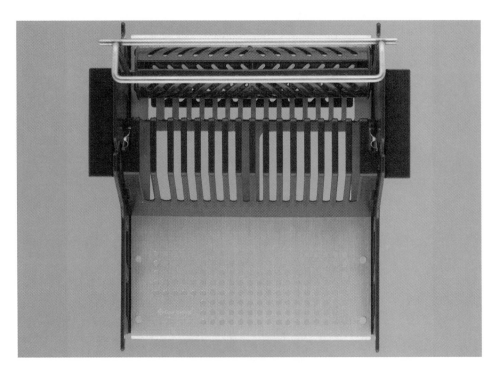

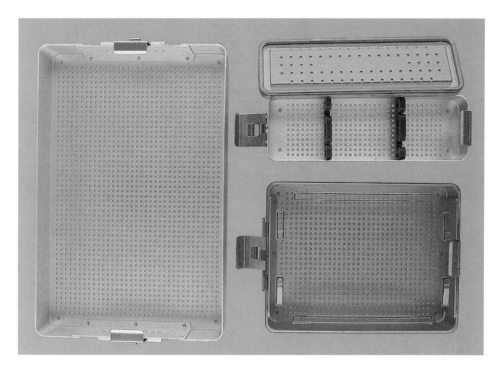

1-3 Various sizes of instrument flash trays.

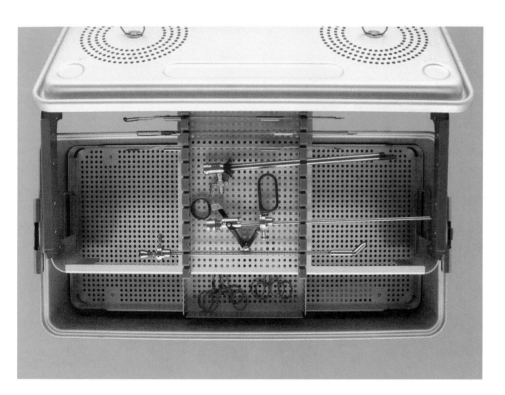

1-4 Large double-tiered sterilizing instrument tray with lid and a few cystoscopy instruments. Steritite™ containers and inserts are compatible with every major sterilization method from steam to gas plasma. (Courtesy Allan and Marcia Frieze, Case Medical, Inc., 65 Railroad Ave., Ridgefield, NJ 07657.)

Unit Two

ABDOMINAL SURGERY

2

Basic Laparotomy Set

2-1 *Left to right,* 2 Masson Mayo Hegar needle holders, 7 inch; 2 Ayer needle holders, 8 inch; 3 Foerster sponge forceps; 2 Mixter hemostatic forceps, long, fine point; 2 Babcock tissue forceps, long; 2 Allis tissue forceps, long; 6 Ochsner hemostatic forceps, long, straight; 4 Mayo Pean hemostatic forceps, long, curved; 6 hemostatic tonsil forceps; 2 Westphal hemostatic forceps; 4 Babcock tissue forceps, short; 4 Allis tissue forceps, short; 8 Crile hemostatic forceps, curved, 6½ inch; 1 Halstead mosquito hemostatic forceps, straight; 6 paper drape clips.

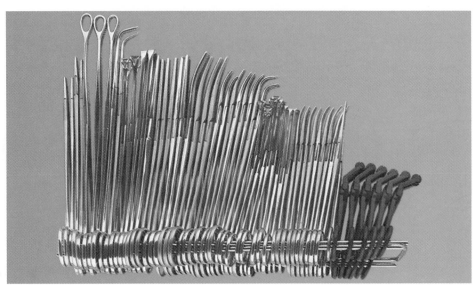

2-2 *Left to right,* 2 Bard Parker knife handles No. 4; 1 Bard Parker knife handle No. 7; 1 Bard Parker knife handle No. 3, long; 1 Mayo dissecting scissors, curved; 2 Mayo dissecting scissors, straight; 1 Metzenbaum dissecting scissors, 7 inch; 1 Snowden-Pencer dissecting scissors, curved; 1 Snowden-Pencer dissecting scissors, straight.

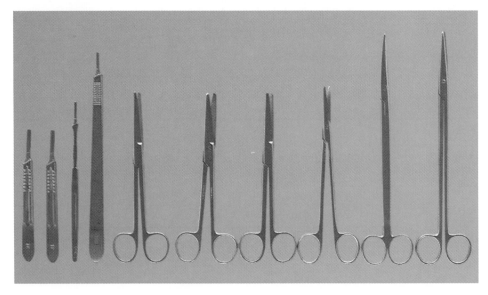

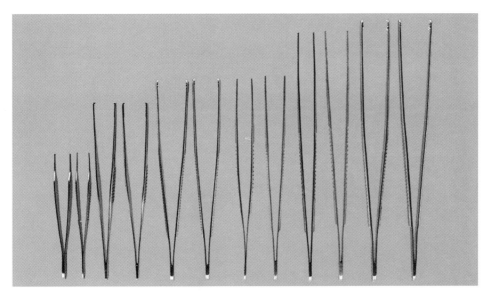

2-3 *Left to right,* 2 Adson tissue forceps with teeth (1 × 2 teeth); 2 Ferris-Smith tissue forceps; 2 Russian tissue forceps, medium; 2 DeBakey Autraugrip tissue forceps, medium; 2 DeBakey Autraugrip tissue forceps, long; 2 Russian tissue forceps, long.

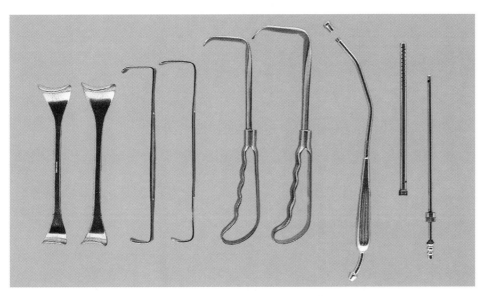

2-4 *Left to right,* 2 Goelet retractors; 2 Army Navy retractors; 1 Richardson retractor, medium; 1 Richardson retractor, large; 1 Yankauer suction tube and tip; 1 Poole abdominal shield and suction tube.

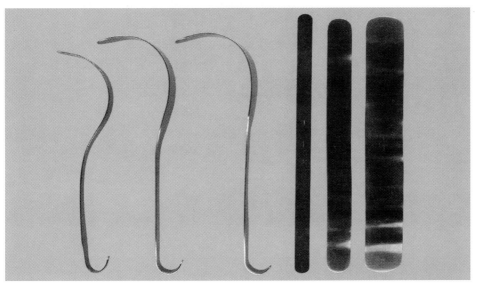

2-5 *Left to right,* Deaver retractors, small, medium, and large; Ochsner malleable retractors, narrow, medium, and wide.

2-6 *Left to right,* Adson tissue forceps and tip (1 × 2); Ferris-Smith tissue forceps and tip; Russian tissue forceps and tip; DeBakey Autraugrip tissue forceps and tip.

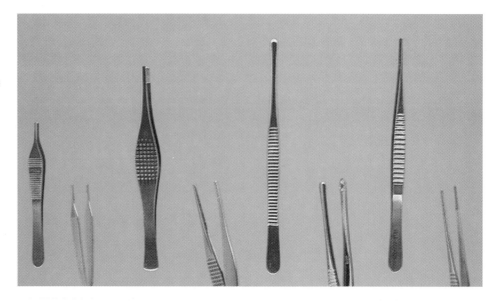

2-7 *Left to right,* Paper drape clip and tip; Halstead mosquito hemostatic forceps, straight, and tip; Halstead hemostatic forceps and tip.

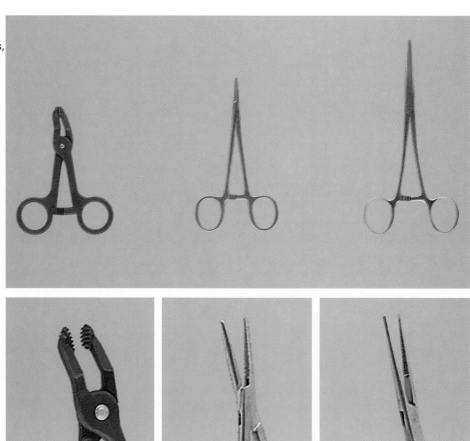

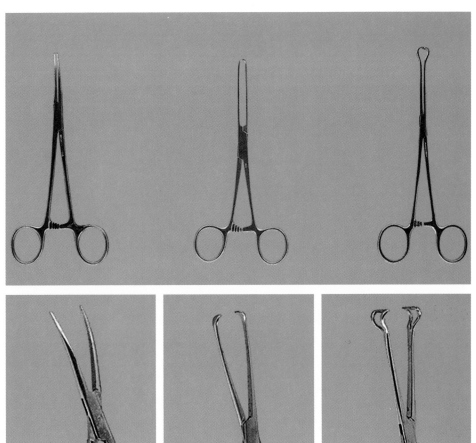

2-8 *Left to right,* Crile hemostatic forceps and tip; Allis tissue forceps and tip; Babcock tissue forceps and tip.

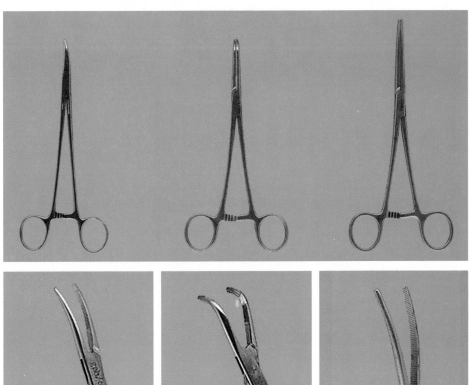

2-9 *Left to right,* Tonsil hemostatic forceps and tip; Westphal hemostatic forceps and tip; Mayo Pean hemostatic forceps and tip.

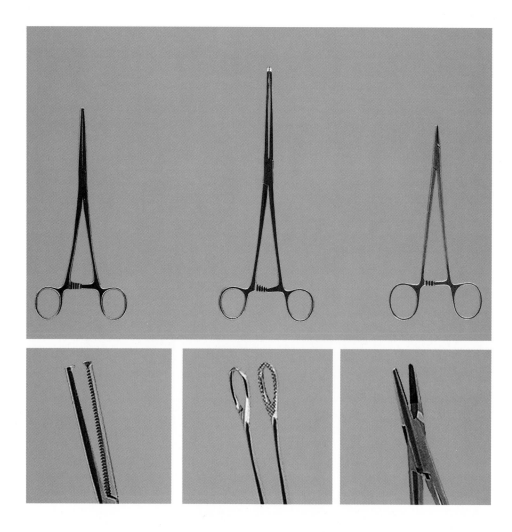

2-10 *Left to right,* Ochsner hemostatic forceps and tip; Foerster sponge forceps and tip; Masson Mayo Hegar needle holder and tip.

3

Long Extra Instruments

ADD TO BASIC LAPAROTOMY SET

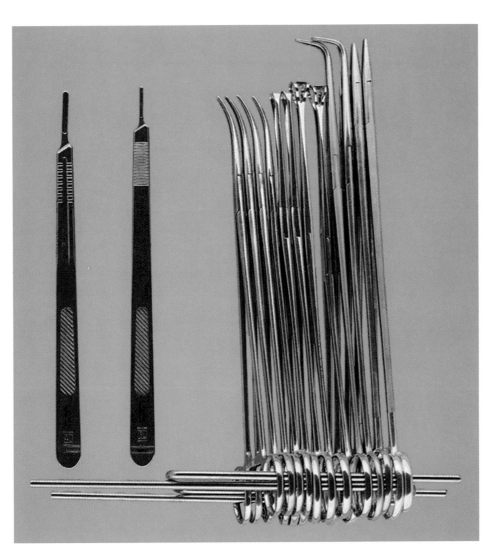

3-1 *Left to right,* 1 Bard Parker knife handle No. 4; 1 Bard Parker knife handle No. 3; 4 tonsil hemostatic forceps, long; 2 Allis tissue forceps, extra long; 2 Babcock tissue forceps, long; 2 Mixter hemostatic forceps, fine tip, extra long; 2 Crile Wood needle holders, 11 inch.

4

Abdominal Self-Retaining Retractors

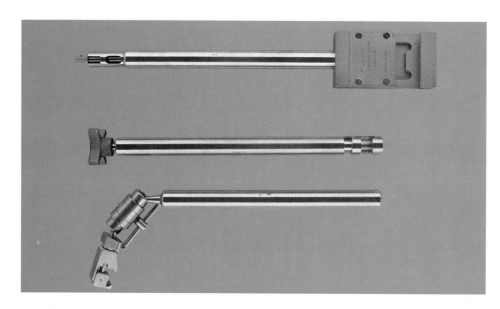

4-1 *Top to bottom,* Bookwalter retractor table post; Bookwalter retractor horizontal bar; Bookwalter retractor horizontal flex bar.

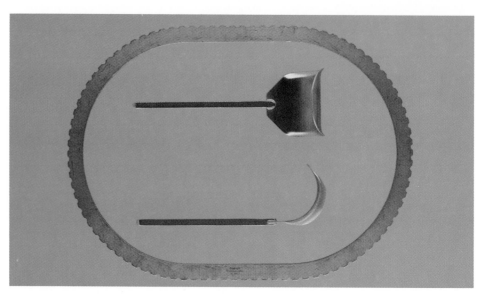

4-2 *Top to bottom,* Bookwalter retractor oval ring, medium; Bookwalter retractor: Balfour blades, second blade, side view.

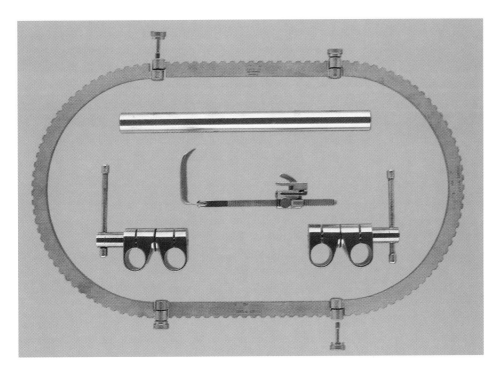

4-3 *Top to bottom,* Bookwalter retractor: segmented parts placed together with 4 locking screws; 2 segmented half circles, medium; 2 segmented straight extensions; 1 vertical extension bar; 1 Kelly retractor blade with ratchet mechanism attached; 2 post couplings.

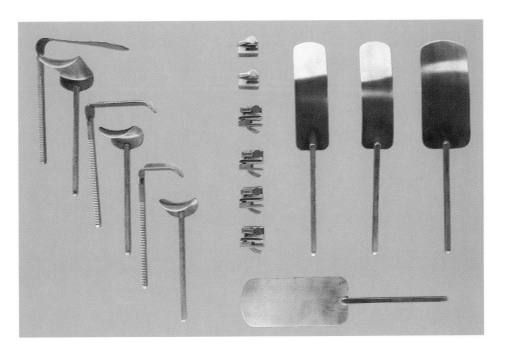

4-4 *Left to right,* 1 Harrington retractor blade; 1 Kelly retractor blade, 2 × 6 inch; 1 Kelly retractor blade, 2 × 4 inch; 1 Kelly retractor blade, 2 × 3 inch; 2 Kelly retractor blades, 2 × 2½ inch; 6 ratchet mechanisms; 2 malleable retractor blades, 2 × 6 inch; 2 malleable retractor blades, 3 × 6 inch.

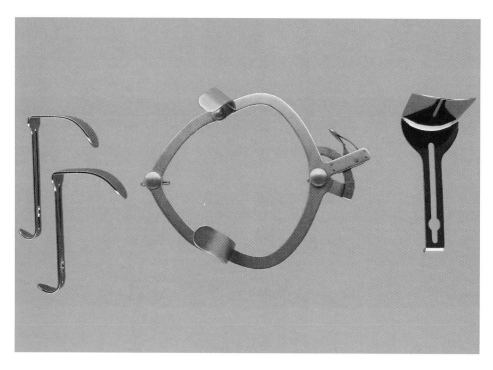

4-5 O'Sullivan-O'Connor retractor with 3 blades.

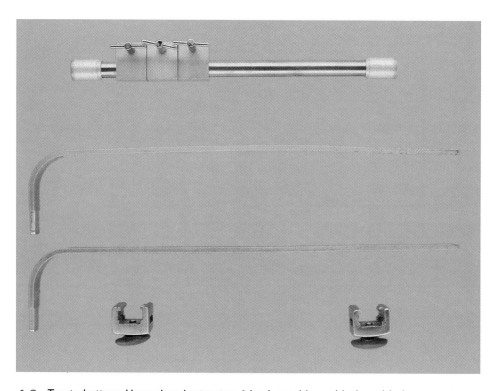

4-6 *Top to bottom,* Upper hand retractor: 1 horizontal bar with three blade supports, 2 vertical arms, and 2 table attachments.

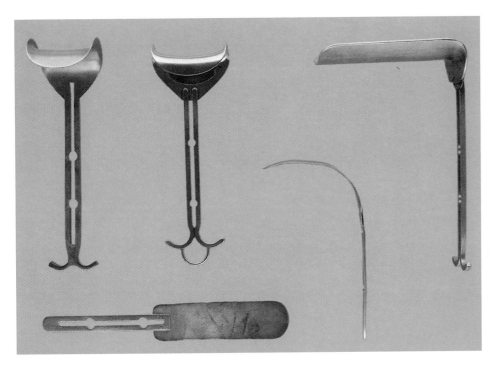

4-7 *Top to bottom, left to right,* Upper hand retractor: 2 Balfour abdominal blades, deep and shallow; 1 Deaver blade, side view; 1 Weinberg blade (modified Joe's Hoe); and 1 malleable blade.

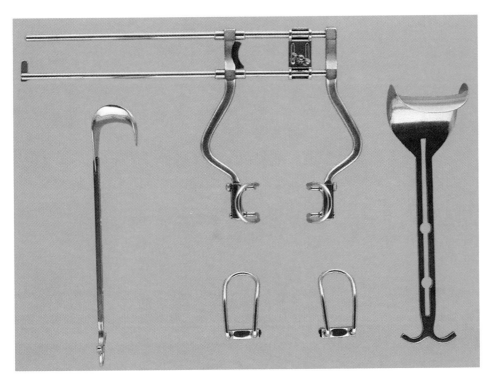

4-8 *Top to bottom, left to right,* Balfour abdominal retractor: retractor frame with 2 detachable shallow fenestrated blades; 1 shallow center blade; 2 deep fenestrated blades; and 1 deep center blade.

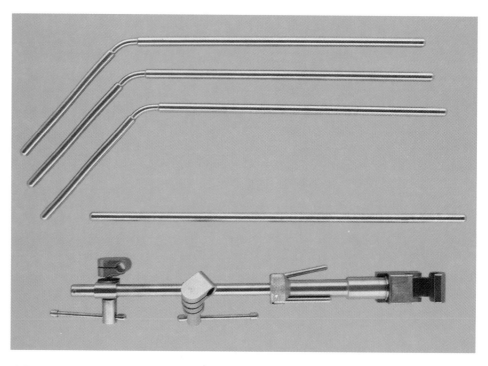

4-9 *Top to bottom,* Thompson retractor. Arms: 3 crossbar elite Thompson angular; 1 extension arm Thompson straight 20 inches; and 1 rail clamp Thompson elite with two joints.

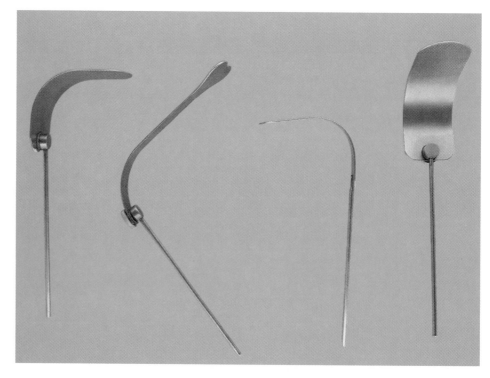

4-10 *Left to right,* Thompson retractor. Rotatable blades: 1 Deaver, medium, side view; 1 Harrington, side view; 1 Deaver, medium (2½ × 5 inch), side view; and 1 Deaver, large, front view.

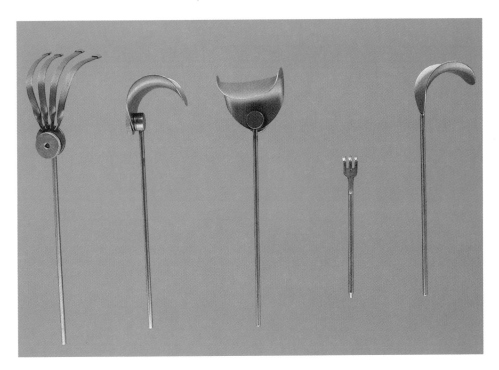

4-11 *Left to right,* Thompson retractor. Rotatable blades: 1 finger malleable; 2 Balfour, side view and back view; 1 rake Murphy, sharp, 3 prong; and 1 Balfour Mayo center (2¾ × 5 inch), side view.

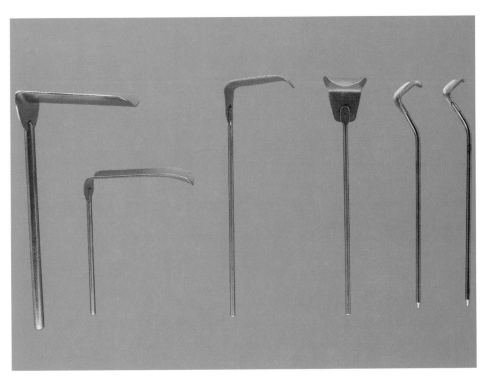

4-12 *Left to right,* Thompson retractor. Rotatable blades: Weinberg (3¼ × 5¼ inch), side view; Richardson (2 × 5 inch), side view; Kelly (2½ × 3 inch), side view; Kelly (2 × 2½ inch), front view; and 2 Richardson carotid (1 × ¼ inch and ¾ × 1 inch), side view.

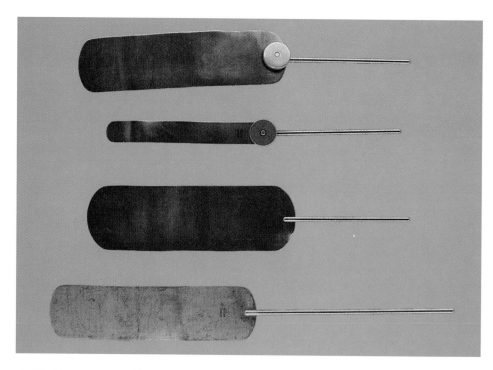

4-13 *Top to bottom,* Thompson retractor. Various sizes of malleable rotatable blades.

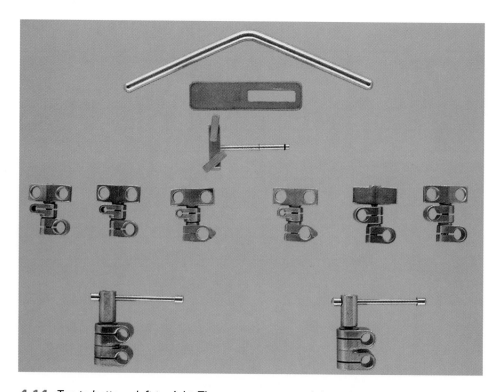

4-14 *Top to bottom, left to right,* Thompson retractor. Joints: 1 extension arm angular, 12 inch; 1 wrench universal; 1 adaptor blade universal; 2 universal (½ × ¼ inch); 2 universal split (½ × ¼ inch); 2 universal (½ × ½ inch); and 2 universal (½ × ½ inch), large.

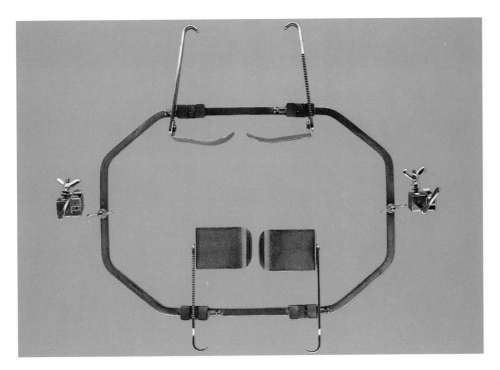

4-15 Wexler retractor: 1 octagon frame; 2 universal joints at each end; and 4 lateral blades: top, side view, and bottom, top view.

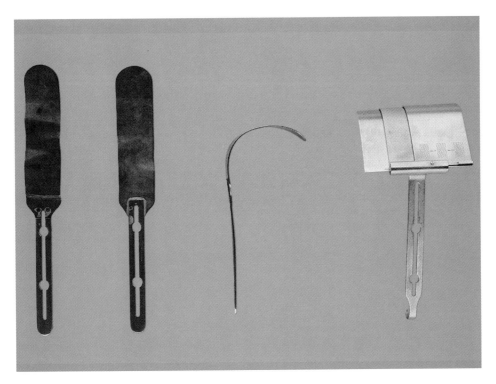

4-16 *Left to right,* Wexler retractor. Blades: 2 malleable; 1 Deaver; and 1 expandable.

5

Hernia or Appendectomy Set

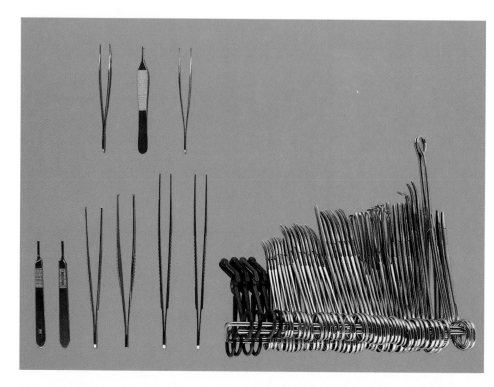

5-1 *Top, left to right,* 1 Brown Adson tissue forceps (7 × 7 teeth); 2 Adson tissue forceps with teeth (1 × 2). *Bottom, left to right,* 2 Bard Parker knife handles, No. 3; 1 Cushing forceps with teeth (1 × 2); 1 Ferris-Smith tissue forceps (1 × 2); 2 DeBakey Autraugrip tissue forceps, medium; 4 paper drape clips; 6 Halstead mosquito hemostatic forceps, curved; 1 Halstead mosquito hemostatic forceps, straight; 8 Crile hemostatic forceps, curved, 5½ inch; 1 Halstead hemostatic forceps, straight; 6 Crile hemostatic forceps, curved, 6½ inch; 4 Allis tissue forceps, short; 4 Babcock tissue forceps, short; 4 Ochsner hemostatic forceps, short; 1 Westphal hemostatic forceps; 2 hemostatic tonsil forceps; 1 Foerster sponge forceps; 2 Masson Mayo Hegar needle holders, 6 inch; 1 Crile Wood needle holder, 6 inch.

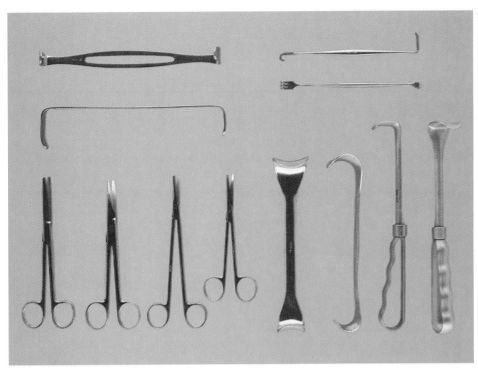

5-2 *Top pairs, left to right,* 2 Army Navy retractors, front view, side view; 2 Miller-Senn retractors, side view, front view. *Bottom, left to right,* 2 Mayo dissecting scissors, straight, curved; 2 Metzenbaum dissecting scissors, 7 inch, 5 inch; 2 Goelet retractors, front view, side view; 2 Richardson retractors, small.

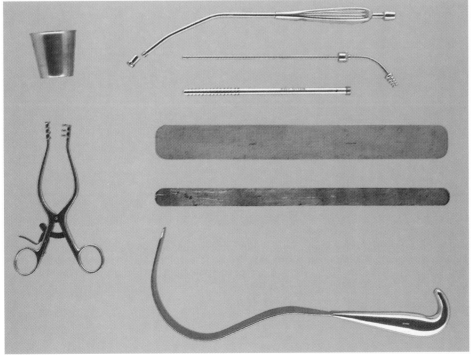

5-3 *Left, top to bottom,* 1 metal medicine cup; 1 Weitlaner retractor, medium. *Right, top to bottom,* 1 Yankauer suction tube with tip; 1 Poole abdominal suction tube with shield; 2 Ochsner malleable retractors, medium, narrow; 1 Deaver retractor, medium.

6

Common Duct Instruments

ADD TO BASIC LAPAROTOMY SET

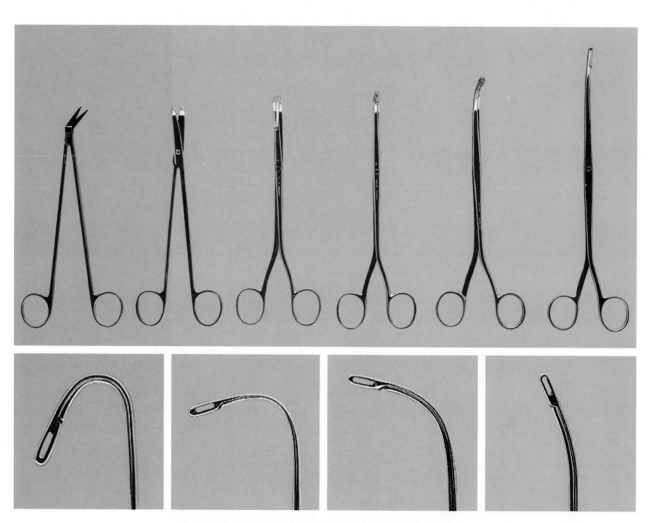

6-1 *Top, left to right,* 1 Potts-Smith cardiovascular scissors, 45-degree angle; 1 Thorek-Feldman scissors; 4 Randall stone forceps, front view (full curved, ¾ curved, ½ curved, and ¼ curved). *Bottom, left to right,* 4 tips of Randall stone forceps, side view (full curved, ¾ curved, ½ curved, and ¼ curved).

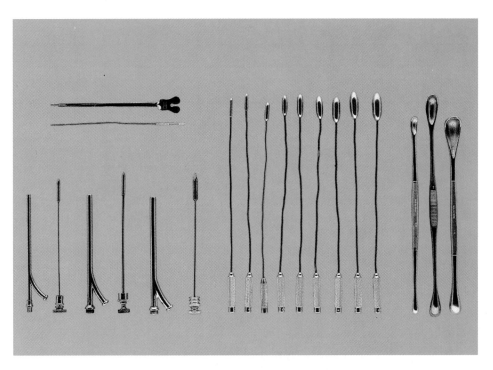

6-2 *Top, left,* 1 grooved director; 1 probe dilator. *Bottom, left to right,* 3 gallbladder trocars with inserts, small, medium, and large; 9 Bake common duct dilators, Nos. 3, 4, 5, 6, 7, 8, 9, 10, 11; 3 Ferguson gallstone scoops, small, medium, and large.

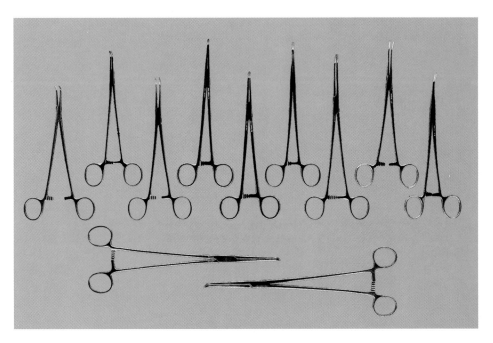

6-3 *Top, left to right,* 2 Adson hemostatic forceps, fine curved; 4 Westphal hemostatic forceps, short; 2 Borge cystic duct catheter clamps, 4 F, 6 F; 1 Mixter hemostatic forceps, fine point, 8½ inch. *Bottom,* 2 Mixter hemostatic forceps, fine point, extra long.

Bowel Resection Instruments

ADD BASIC LAPAROTOMY SET AND SELF-RETAINING RETRACTOR

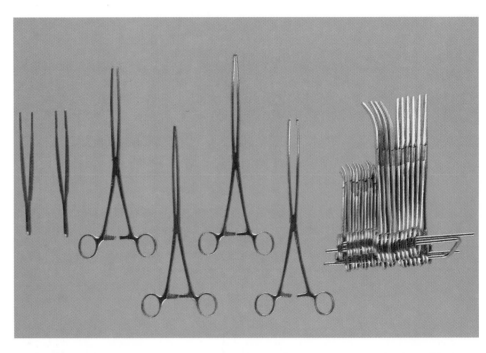

7-1 *Left to right,* 2 DeBakey Autraugrip tissue forceps, short; 2 Doyen intestinal forceps, straight; 2 Doyen intestinal forceps, curved; 12 Halstead mosquito hemostatic forceps, curved; 4 Carmalt hemostatic forceps, long, curved; 6 Carmalt hemostatic forceps, long, straight.

Hysterectomy Instruments

ADD BASIC LAPAROTOMY SET

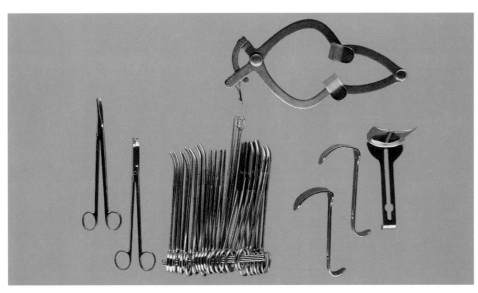

8-1 *Top, left,* 1 O'Sullivan-O'Connor retractor body. *Bottom, left to right,* 1 Mayo dissecting scissors, curved, 9 inch; 1 Jorgenson dissecting scissors, curved, 9 inch; 4 Ochsner hemostatic forceps, 8 inch; 2 Heaney hysterectomy forceps, single tooth; 2 Heaney Ballentine hysterectomy forceps, single tooth; 4 Ochsner hemostatic forceps, 8 inch; 1 Schroeder uterine tenaculum forceps, single tooth; 1 Skene uterine vulsellum forceps, straight, double tooth; 2 Masterson clamps, straight; 2 Masterson clamps, curved; 2 Heaney needle holders.

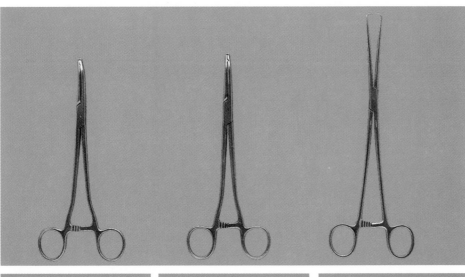

8-2 *Left to right,* 1 Heaney hysterectomy forceps, single tooth, and tip; 1 Heaney Ballentine hysterectomy forceps, single tooth, and tip; 1 Schroeder uterine tenaculum forceps, single tooth; and tip of Skene uterine vulsellum forceps, straight, double tooth.

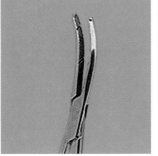
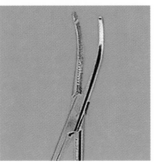
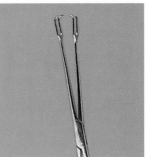

8-3 *Left to right,*
A, 1 Jorgenson dissecting scissors tip, curved; **B**, 1 Masterson clamp, straight, and tip; **C**, 1 Masterson clamp, curved, and tip; **D**, 1 Heaney needle holder and tip; .

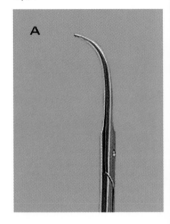

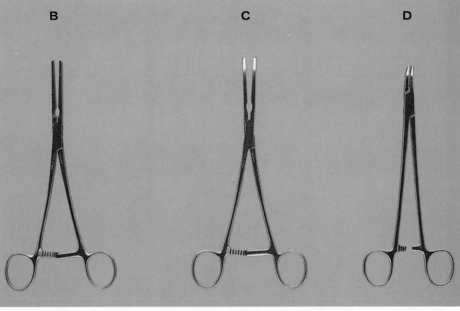

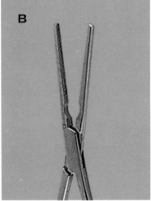

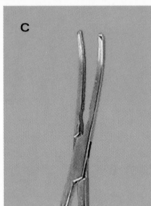

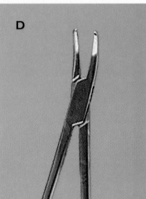

9

Microtuboplasty Instruments

ADD BASIC LAPAROTOMY SET AND SELF-RETAINING RETRACTOR

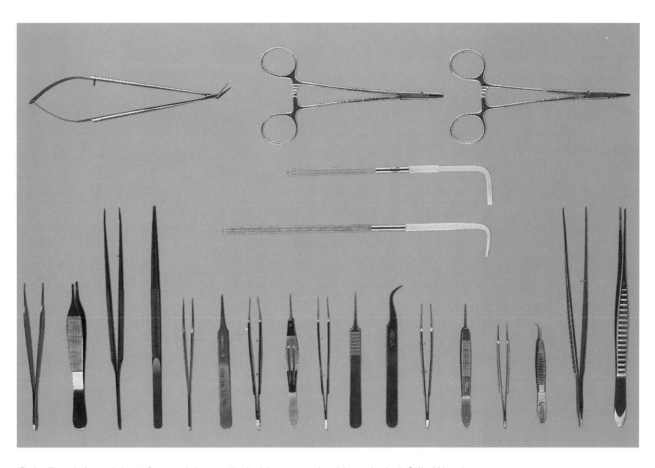

9-1 *Top, left to right,* 1 Castroviejo needle holder, curved, without lock; 2 Crile Wood needle holders, 6 inch; 2 Swolin Teflon angled rods on handles, 1 mm, 3.5 mm. *Bottom, left to right,* 2 Brown Adson tissue forceps (7 × 7), front view, side view; 2 titanium tying forceps, front view, side view; 3 jeweler's forceps No. 3, front view, side view, front view; 2 Castroviejo suturing forceps, 0.12 mm, with tying platforms, side view, front view; 1 Castroviejo suturing forceps, 0.5mm, with tying platforms; 1 jeweler's forceps, curved, side view; 2 Harms tying forceps without teeth, front view, side view; 1 McPherson tying forceps, straight, front view; 1 Kelman-McPherson tying forceps, curved, side view; 2 Cushing thumb forceps, front view, side view.

9-2 *Left to right,*
A, Brown Adson tissue forceps (7 × 7) and tip; **B**, Castroviejo suturing forceps, 0.12 mm, and tip; **C**, jeweler's forceps and tip; **D**, McPherson tying forceps, straight; **E**, Kelman-McPherson tying forceps tip, curved; **F**, jeweler's forceps tip, curved.

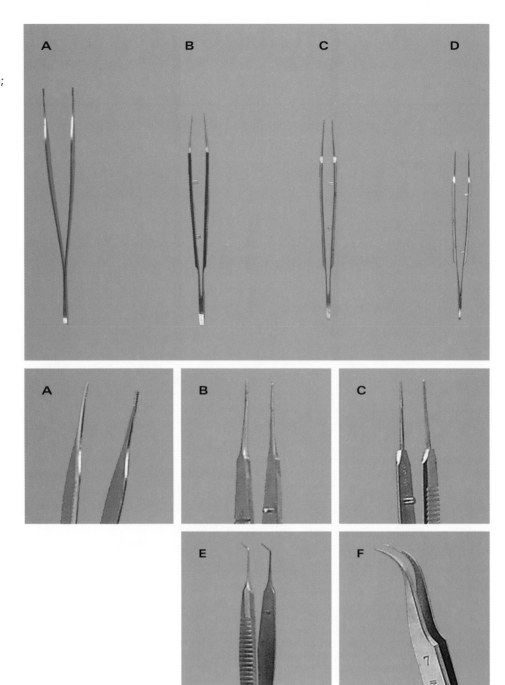

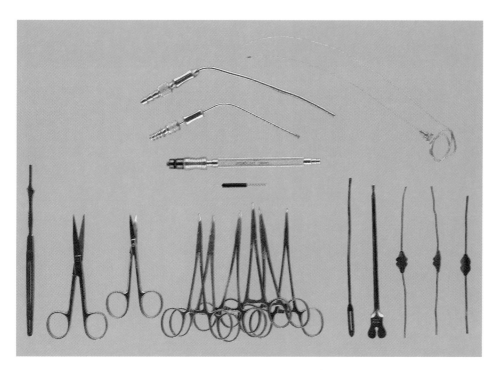

9-3 *Top to bottom,* 2 Frazier suction tubes with stylets, 11 Fr and 8 Fr; 1 Gomel irrigator; 1 nondisposable needle electrode, $7/8$ inch. *Bottom, left to right,* 1 Bard Parker knife handle, No. 7; 2 plastic scissors, straight and curved; 6 Halstead mosquito hemostatic forceps, curved, delicate; 1 probe dilator; 1 grooved director; 3 Bowman (lacrymal) probes, 00-0, 1-2, 3-4.

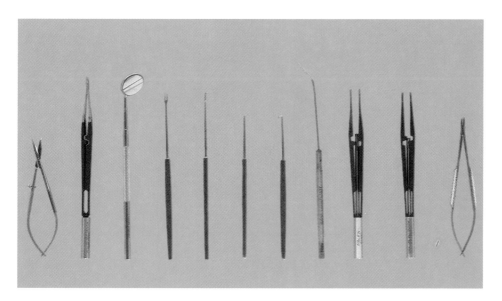

9-4 *Left to right,* 1 Vannas capsulotomy scissors; 1 Vannas microscissors, curved; 1 front surface dental mirror (DMS-5 rhodium only); 2 Guthrie hooks, double, sharp; 2 Gillies converse skin hooks, single; 1 microprobe; 1 Storz microforceps with teeth; 1 Storz microforceps without teeth; 1 Storz microscissors.

9-5 *Left to right,* **A,** Guthrie hook, double, sharp, and tip; **B,** Gillies converse skin hook, single, and tip; **C,** Storz microforceps, without teeth, and tip with teeth; **D,** titanium tying forceps, and tip.

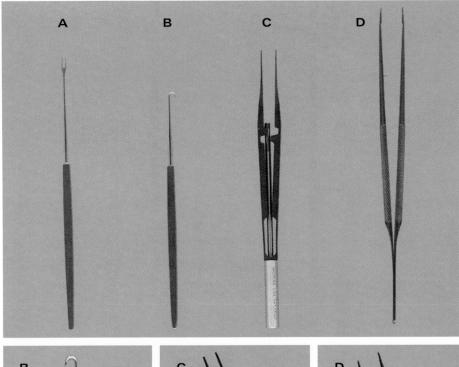

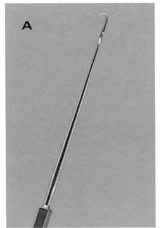

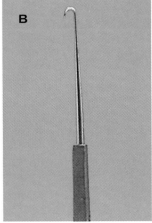

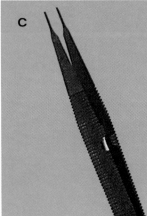

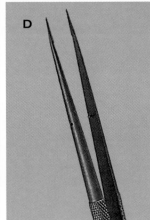

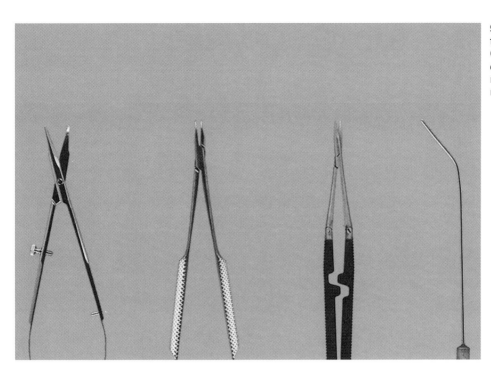

9-6 *Left to right,* Westcott tenotomy scissors, tip; Castroviejo needle holder, curved, tip; Vannas microscissors, curved, tip; microprobe, tip.

10

Nephrectomy and Ureteroplasty Instruments

ADD BASIC LAPAROTOMY SET AND SELF-RETAINING RETRACTOR

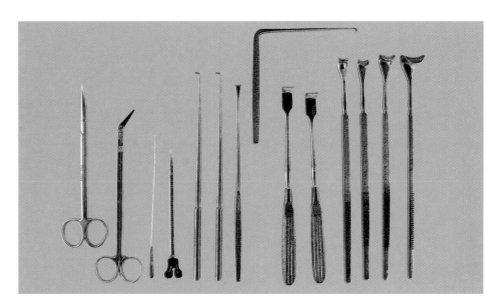

10-1 *Left to right,* 1 Lincoln Metzenbaum scissors, narrow dissecting tip; 1 Potts-Smith cardiovascular scissors, 45-degree angle; 1 probe dilator; 1 grooved director; 2 Hoen nerve hooks; 2 Love nerve retractors, straight, 90-degree angle; 2 Little retractors, medium; 4 Gil-Vernet retractors, assorted sizes.

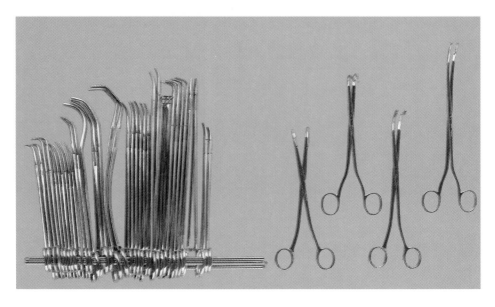

10-2 *Left to right,* 4 Westphal hemostatic forceps; 6 hemostatic tonsil forceps; 2 Adson hemostatic forceps, fine curved; 1 Mayo Guyon kidney forceps; 2 Herrick kidney forceps; 2 Satinsky (vena cava) forceps; 6 hemostatic tonsil forceps, 9$\frac{1}{2}$ inch; 2 hemostatic tonsil forceps, 10$\frac{1}{2}$ inch; 2 Babcock tissue forceps, extra long; 4 Mixter hemostatic forceps, 10$\frac{1}{2}$ inch, fine tip; 2 Ayer needle holders, extra long; 2 Heaney needle holders, long; 4 Randall stone forceps: full curve, $\frac{3}{4}$ curve, $\frac{1}{2}$ curve, and $\frac{1}{4}$ curve.

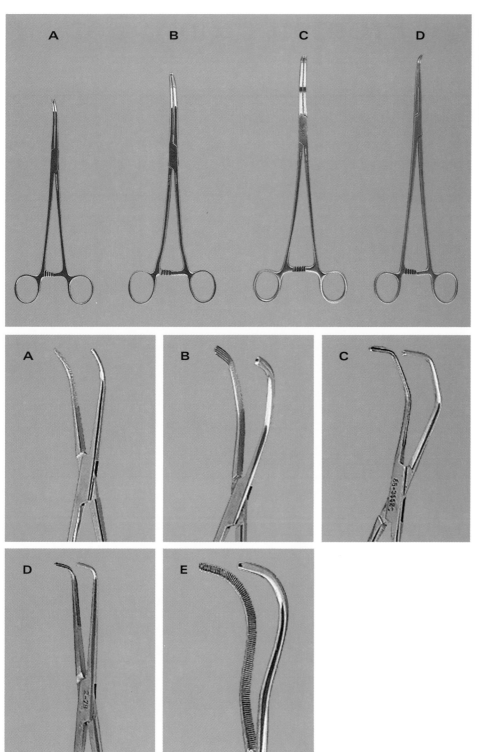

10-3 *Left to right,* **A,** Adson hemostatic forceps, fine tip, and tip; **B,** Herrick kidney forceps, and tip; **C,** Satinsky (vena cava) forceps and tip; **D,** Mixter hemostatic forceps, 10½ inch, fine tip, and tip; **E,** Mayo Guyon kidney forceps, tip.

11

Radical Prostatectomy Set

MAY ADD ADDITIONAL RETRACTORS

11-1 *Top,* 1 Poole abdominal suction tube and shield. *Left to right,* 2 Yankauer suction tubes and tips; 6 paper drape clips; 4 Halstead mosquito hemostatic forceps, curved; 4 Halstead mosquito hemostatic forceps, straight; 1 Halstead hemostatic forceps; 6 Crile hemostatic forceps, $6^{1}/_{2}$ inch; 4 hemostatic tonsil forceps; 2 Mayo Pean hemostatic forceps, curved; 2 Allis tissue forceps, medium; 1 Babcock tissue forceps, medium; 4 Ochsner hemostatic forceps, straight, long jaw; 6 Mixter hemostatic forceps, 9 inch; 6 hemostatic tonsil forceps, long; 4 Allis tissue forceps, extra long, curved; 4 Mixter hemostatic forceps, extra long; 3 Foerster sponge forceps; 2 Crile Wood needle holders, 7 inch; 2 Crile Wood needle holders, 8 inch; 2 Masson Mayo Hegar needle holders, 12 inch.

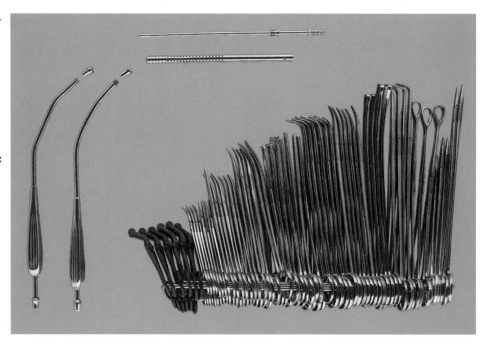

11-2 *Left to right,* 2 Adson tissue forceps (1 × 2); 2 Ferris-Smith tissue forceps (1 × 2); 2 Russian tissue forceps; 2 thumb tissue forceps with teeth (1 × 2), long; 2 DeBakey Autraugrip tissue forceps, long; 2 DeBakey Autraugrip tissue forceps, extra long.

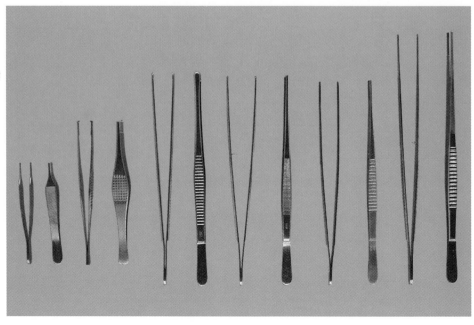

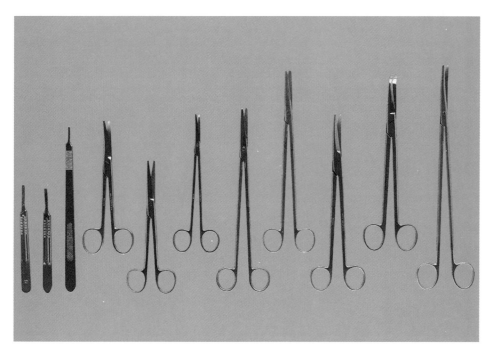

11-3 *Left to right,* 2 Bard Parker knife handles, No. 4; 1 Bard Parker knife handle, No. 3, long; 2 Mayo dissecting scissors, curved and straight; 2 Metzenbaum dissecting scissors, 7 inch and extra long; 2 Snowden-Pencer scissors, straight and curved; 1 Jorgenson dissecting scissors; 1 Mayo dissecting scissors, long, curved.

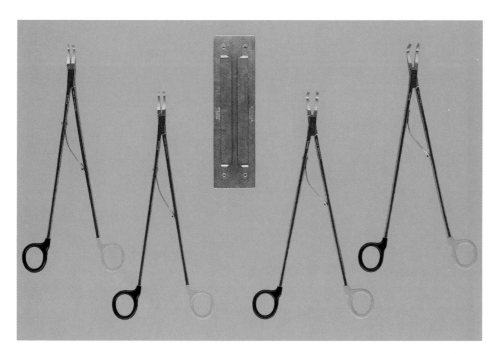

11-4 *Left to right,* 2 Samuels hemoclip-applying forceps, medium; 1 Hemoclip cartridge base for hemoclips; 2 Samuels hemoclip-applying forceps, large.

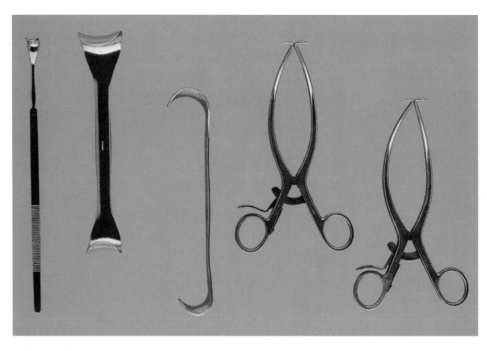

11-5 *Left to right,* 1 Gil-Vernet retractor; 2 Goelet retractors, front view, side view; 2 Gelpi retractors.

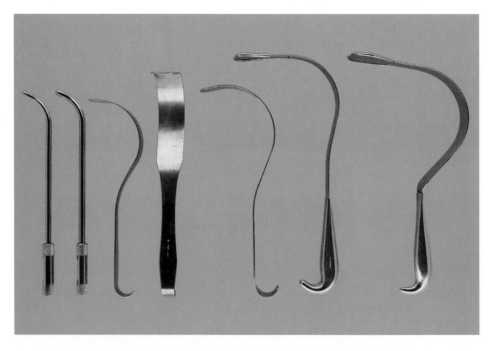

11-6 *Left to right,* 2 Greenwald suture guides, 24 Fr, 28 Fr; 3 Deaver retractors: narrow, side view; medium, front view; and wide, side view; 2 Harrington splanchnic retractors, small and large.

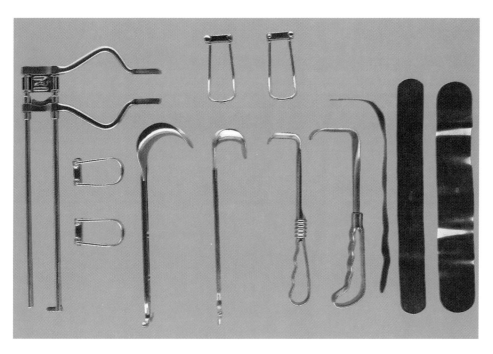

11-7 *Top,* 2 Balfour abdominal retractor fenestrated blades, large. *Left to right,* 1 Balfour abdominal retractor frame; 2 Balfour abdominal retractor fenestrated blades, small; 2 Balfour abdominal retractor center blades, large, small; 2 Richardson retractors, medium, large; 3 Ochsner malleable retractors, narrow (side view), medium, large.

Unit Three

GENERAL SURGERY

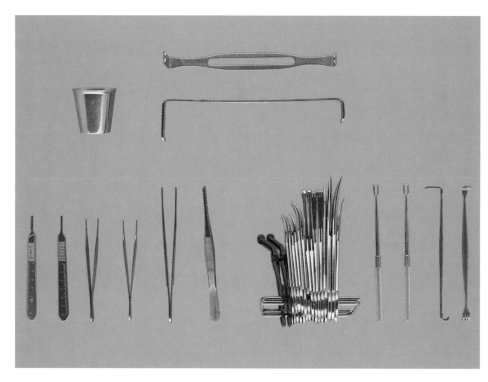

12-1 *Top, left to right,* 1 medicine cup, metal; 2 Army Navy retractors, front view, side view. *Bottom, left to right,* 2 Bard Parker knife handles, No. 3; 1 Adson tissue forceps (1 × 2); 1 Brown Adson tissue forceps (7 × 7); 2 DeBakey Autraugrip tissue forceps, short; 2 paper drape clips; 4 Halstead mosquito hemostatic forceps, curved; 2 Crile hemostatic forceps, 5¹/₂ inch; 2 Allis tissue forceps; 2 Lahey thyroid tenaculums; 1 Crile Wood needle holder, 6 inch; 2 Mayo dissecting scissors, straight, curved; 1 Metzenbaum dissecting scissors, 5 inch; 2 Joseph skin hooks, double; 2 Miller-Senn retractors, side view, front view.

Radical Dissecting Set

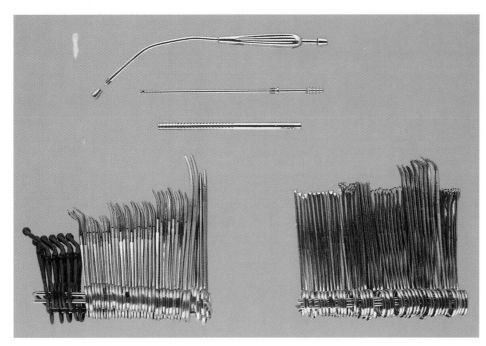

13-1 *Top to bottom,* Yankauer suction tube and tip; Poole abdominal suction tube and shield. *Bottom, left to right,* 6 paper drape clips; 2 Backhaus towel forceps; 8 Halstead mosquito hemostatic forceps, curved; 12 Crile hemostatic forceps, 5¹/₂ inch; 8 Crile hemostatic forceps, 6¹/₂ inch; 2 Mayo Pean hemostatic forceps, long; 2 Johnson needle holders, delicate jaw, 5 inch; 2 Crile Wood needle holders, 7 inch; 12 Allis tissue forceps; 4 Babcock tissue forceps; 4 Ochsner hemostatic forceps, straight, short; 8 Adair breast forceps, short; 4 hemostatic tonsil forceps; 4 Westphal hemostatic forceps; 4 Lahey thyroid tenaculums.

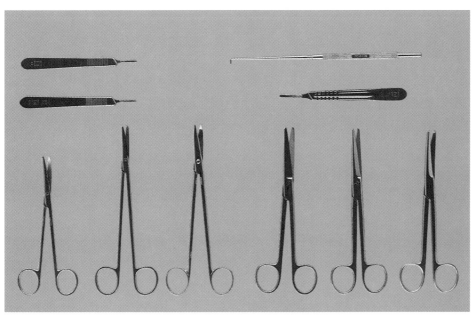

13-2 *Top, left to right,* 2 Bard Parker knife handles, No. 3; Hoen nerve hook; 1 Bard Parker knife handle, No. 4. *Bottom, left to right,* 2 Metzenbaum dissecting scissors, 5 inch, 6 inch; 1 Prince-Metzenbaum dissecting scissors; Mayo dissecting scissors, 2 straight, 1 curved.

13-3 *Left to right,* 2 Adson tissue forceps with teeth (1 × 2), front view, side view; 2 Brown Adson tissue forceps (7 × 7), front view, side view; 1 Adson tissue forceps without teeth, front view; 2 DeBakey Autraugrip tissue forceps, short; 2 Hayes Martin tissue forceps, short; 2 DeBakey Autraugrip tissue forceps, medium.

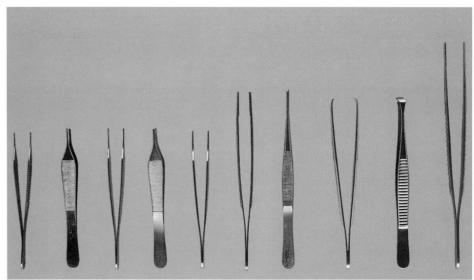

13-4 *Left to right,* 2 Richardson retractors, small, medium; 2 Volkmann retractors, 6 prong, sharp, front view, side view; 2 Volkmann retractors, 6 prong, dull, front view, side view; 2 Volkmann retractors, 4 prong, dull, front view, side view; 2 Volkmann retractors, 4 prong, sharp, front view, side view.

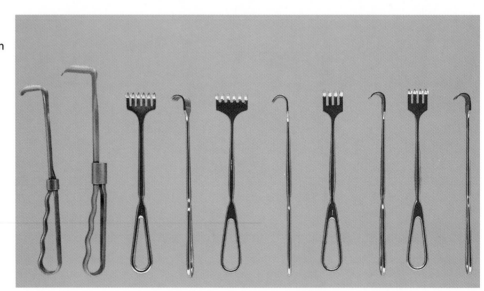

13-5 *Left to right,* 2 Army Navy retractors, side view, front view; 2 Langenbeck retractors, side view, front view; 2 Green goiter retractors, side view, front view; 2 Cushing vein retractors, side view, front view; 2 Miller-Senn retractors, side view, front view.

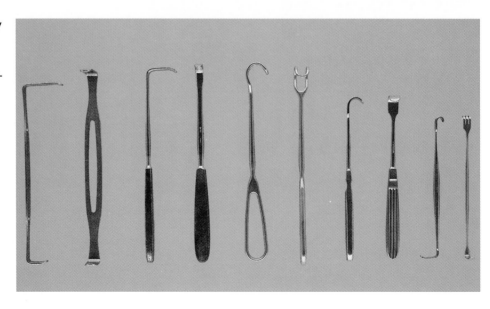

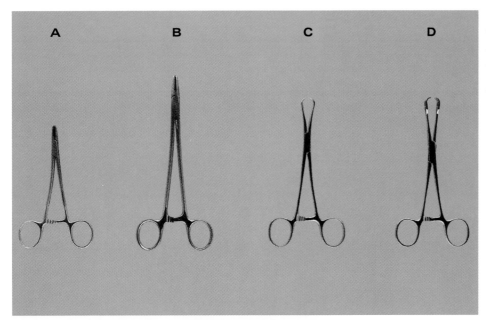

13-6 *Left to right,* **A,** Johnson needle holder, delicate jaw, and tip; **B,** Crile Wood needle holder and tip; **C,** Adair breast forceps and tip; **D,** Lahey thyroid forceps and tip.

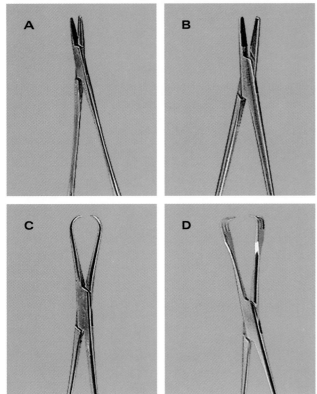

14

Skin Staplers

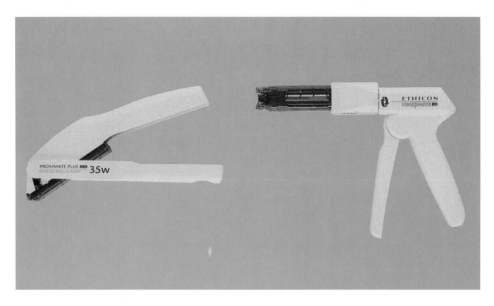

14-1 *Left to right,* Skin staplers, disposable, fixed head and rotating head.

Vascular Access for Therapy

Add 2 Bard Parker knife handles, No. 3; 1 Adson tissue forceps with teeth (1 × 2); 1 Metzenbaum dissecting scissors, 5 inch; 3 Halstead mosquito hemostatic forceps, curved; 1 Mayo dissecting scissors, straight; 2 Miller-Senn retractors; 1 Johnson needle holder; 1 tunneling instrument (Takahashi nasal forceps, straight, or Pratt dilators, No. 13-15, No. 17-19). Central venous ports and catheters are placed in subclavian or internal jugular veins. Add central venous port or catheter kit. Peripheral venous ports (PAS) are placed in the basilic or cephalic veins. Add peripheral venous port kit and catheter finder. Delete tunneling instrument.

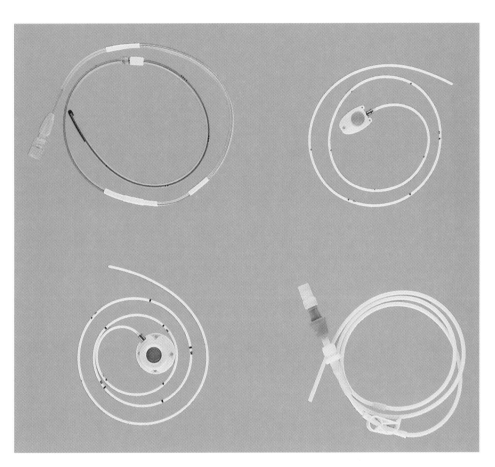

15-1 *Top, left to right,* Groshong catheter for central venous access; peripheral venous port with catheter attached. *Bottom, left to right,* Central venous port with catheter attached; Hickman catheter for central venous access.

Tracheotomy Set

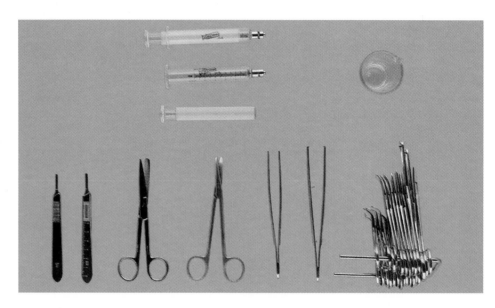

16-1 *Top, left to right,* 2 glass 10 ml syringes, together and separate; 1 glass medicine cup. *Bottom, left to right,* 2 Bard Parker knife handles, No. 3; 1 plastic suture scissors, 5½ inch; 1 Metzenbaum dissecting scissors, 5 inch; 2 thumb tissue forceps, without teeth, with teeth (1 × 2); 4 Backhaus towel clips; 6 Halstead mosquito hemostatic forceps, 3 curved, 3 straight; 2 Allis tissue forceps; 1 Johnson needle holder, 5 inch.

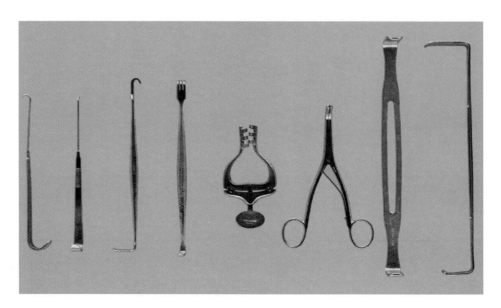

16-2 *Left to right,* 2 tracheal hooks, side view, front view; 2 Miller-Senn retractors, side view, front view; 1 articulated mastoid retractor; 1 Trousseau-Jackson tracheal dilator; 2 Army Navy retractors, front view, side view.

ENDOSCOPIC SURGERY

Laparoscope

MANY OF THE ENDOSCOPIC INSTRUMENTS CAN BE USED INTERCHANGEABLY WITHIN THE VARIOUS ENDOSCOPIC SPECIALITIES. INTERCHANGEABLE TERMS: OBTURATOR—TROCAR; CANNULA—PORT OR SLEEVE.

17-1 *Top to bottom,* Laparoscope and fiberoptic light cord.

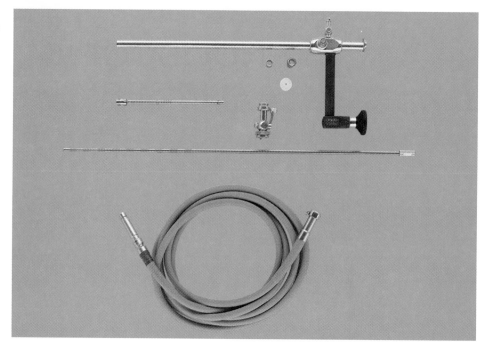

17-2 *Top to bottom,* Nondisposable laparoscopic lens: 0 degree 5 mm, 25 degree 5 mm, 50 degree 5 mm, 25 degree 10 mm, and 50 degree 10 mm.

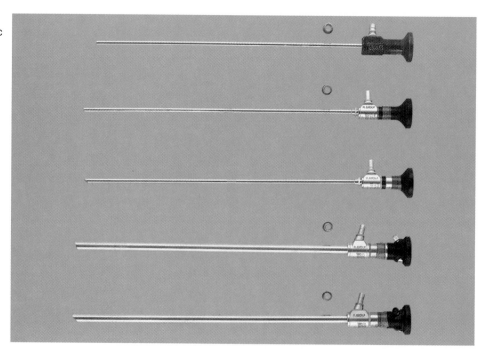

Minor Instrument Set

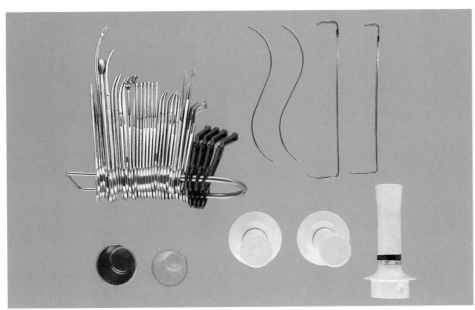

18-1 *Top, left to right,* 1 Crile Wood needle holder, 6 inch; 2 Johnson needle holder, 5 inch; 1 Randall stone forceps, 1/4 curve; 1 stone extractor forceps; 1 Mayo Pean hemostatic forceps, curved; 4 Crile hemostatic forceps, 6 1/2 inch; 2 Babcock tissue forceps; 6 Allis tissue forceps; 4 Crile hemostatic forceps, 5 1/2 inch; 2 Ochsner hemostatic forceps, short; 1 Mayo dissecting scissors, straight; 1 Metzenbaum dissecting scissors; 2 Backhaus towel clips; 4 paper drape clips; 2 S retractors, side view; 2 Army Navy retractors, side view. *Bottom, left to right,* 2 medicine cups, metal, glass; 3 light handles, 2 upright, 1 side view.

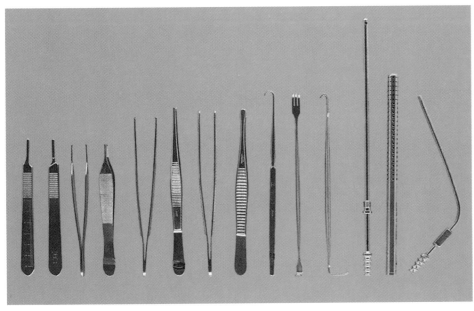

18-2 *Left to right,* 2 Bard Parker knife handles, No. 3; 2 Adson tissue forceps with teeth (1 × 2); 2 thumb tissue forceps without teeth; 2 Russian tissue forceps; 1 tracheal hook; 2 Senn-Kanavel retractors, front view, side view; 1 Poole abdominal suction tube and shield; 1 Frazier suction tube, 9 Fr.

18-3 *Left to right,* Backhaus towel clips and tip; Randall stone forceps, $1/4$ curve; Jarit stone extractor forceps and tip.

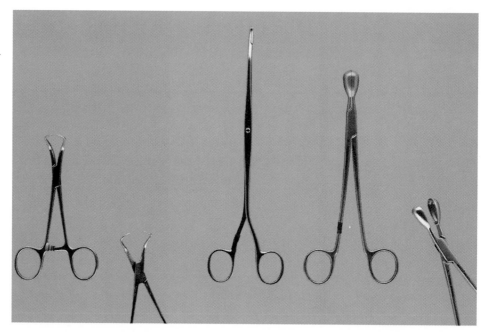

19

Laparoscopic Cholecystectomy Set

ADD LAPAROSCOPE, LIGHT CORD, AND MINOR INSTRUMENT SET

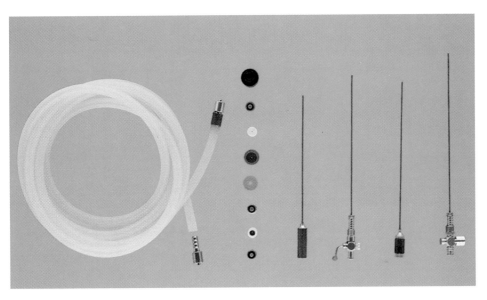

19-1 *Left to right,* 1 Silastic (silicone elastomer) tubing, 8 foot long, with male Luer-Lok; 1 male Luer-Lok adapter; 2 gray nipples with small hole; 3 port caps; 1 red rubber cap with pinhole; 1 gray rubber cap with 3 mm hole; 1 Verres needle, medium; 1 Verres needle stylet, medium; 1 Verres needle, long; 1 Verres needle stylet, long.

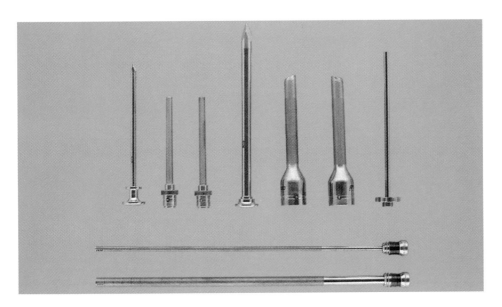

19-2 *Top, left to right,* 1 Applied obturator, 5 mm, 100 mm length; 2 Applied cannulas, 5 mm, 100 mm length; 1 Applied obturator, 10 mm, 100 mm length; 2 Applied cannulas, 10 mm, 100 mm length; 1 Nezhat Dorsey plug. *Bottom, top to bottom,* 2 Nezhat suction tips, 5 mm, 10 mm.

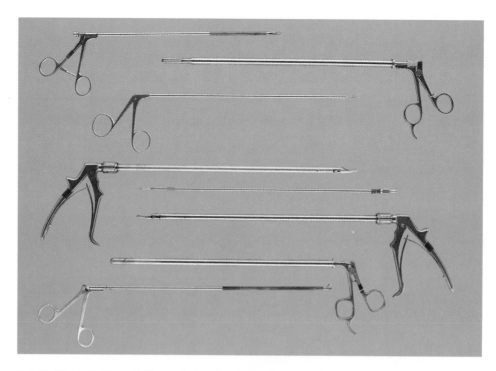

19-3 *Top to bottom,* 1 Olsen cholangio clamp, 5 mm; 1 claw grasper, 10 mm; 1 microdissector, 5 mm; 1 medium/large ligaclip appliers with roticulating shaft; 1 aspiration needle, 5 mm; 1 medium/large ligaclip appliers with roticulating shaft; 1 large spring-loaded double-spoon grasper; 1 Hook scissors, 5 mm.

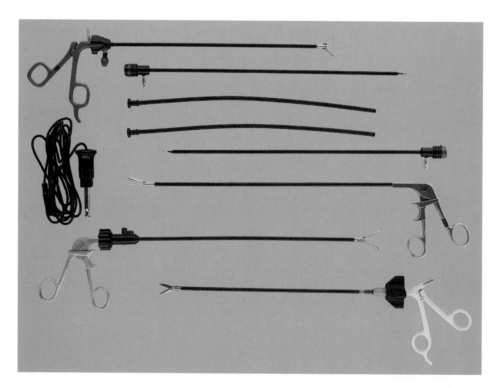

19-4 *Left,* Monopolar cord. *Top to bottom,* 1 Maryland dissector, curved tip, 5 mm; 1 Nezhat Dorsey spatula, 5 mm; 2 Nezhat Dorsey sleeves; 1 Nezhat Dorsey insulated L-hook probe, 5 mm; 1 atraumatic gallbladder grasper, 5 mm; 1 aggressive grasper with teeth, 5 mm; 1 monopolar Metzenbaum scissors, 5 mm.

LAPAROSCOPIC CHOLECYSTECTOMY

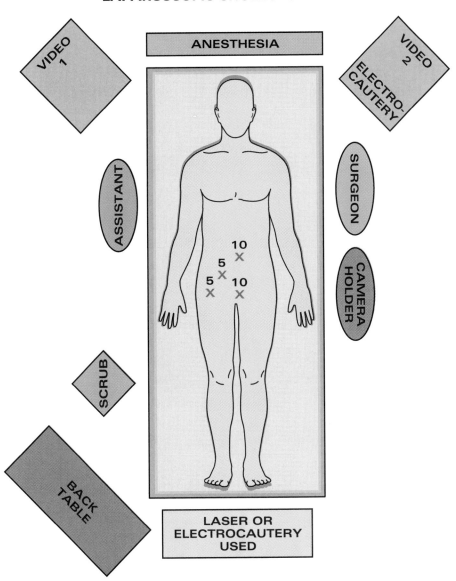

19-5 Cholecystectomy.

Laparoscopic Advanced Set

ADD LAPAROSCOPE, LIGHT CORD, AND MINOR INSTRUMENT SET. USED FOR DIAGNOSTIC TO ADVANCED PROCEDURES.

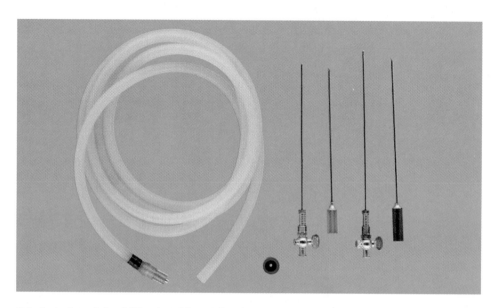

20-1 *Left to right,* 1 Silastic tubing, 8 foot long, with one male Luer-Lok end; 1 rubber cap; 1 Verres needle stylet, medium; 1 Verres needle, medium; 1 Verres needle stylet, long; 1 Verres needle, long.

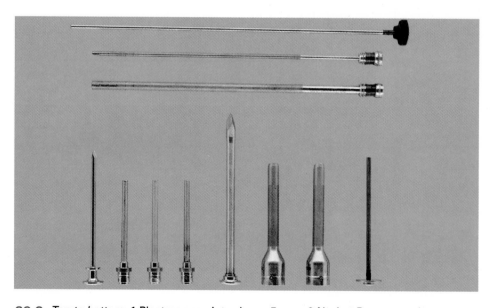

20-2 *Top to bottom,* 1 Pleatman sac introducer, 5 mm; 2 Nezhat Dorsey suction cannulas, 5 mm, 10 mm. *Left to right,* 1 Applied obturator, 5 mm, 100 mm length; 3 Applied cannulas, 5 mm, 100 mm length; 1 Applied obturator, 10 mm, 100 mm length; 2 Applied cannulas, 10 mm, 100 mm length; 1 endoscopic loop introducer, 5 mm.

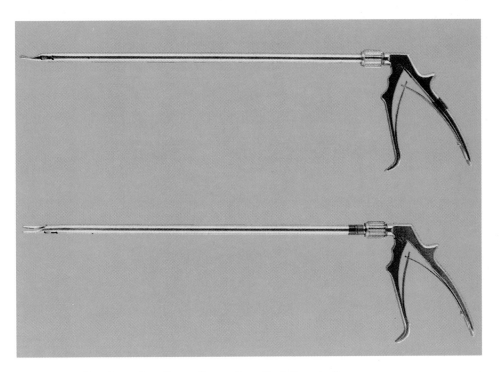

20-3 2 medium/large ligaclip appliers with roticulating shaft.

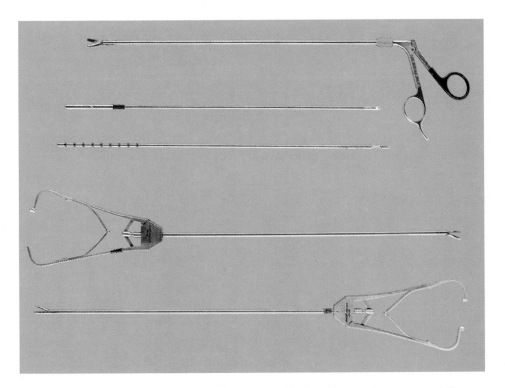

20-4 *Top to bottom,* 1 ligature scissors, 5 mm; 1 Marlow knot pusher, open end, 5 mm;
1 Ranfac knot pusher, closed end, 5 mm; 2 locking curved needle holders, 5 mm.

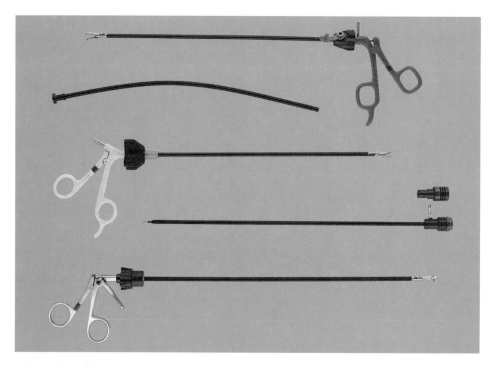

20-5 *Top to bottom,* 1 Maryland dissector, curved tip, 5 mm; 1 Nezhat Dorsey sheath, 5 mm; 1 monopolar Metzenbaum scissors, 5 mm; 1 Nezhat Dorsey plug; 1 Nezhat Dorsey insulated L-hook probe, 5 mm; 1 Swanstrom Babcock with lock, 5 mm.

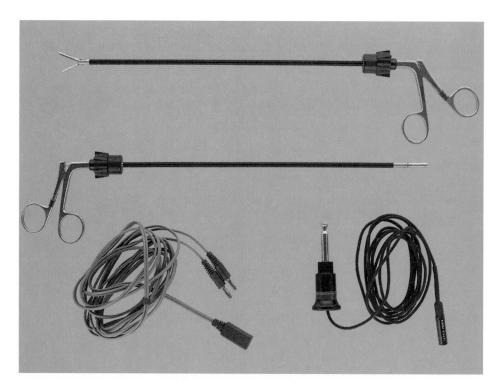

20-6 *Top to bottom,* 2 Hunter bowel graspers, 5 mm (Glassman type); 1 Everest bipolar cord; 1 monopolar cord.

Laparoscopic Advanced Extra Instruments

GYNECOLOGY EXTRAS. SIGMOID AND LOW ANTERIOR COLON RESECTIONS (SEE FIGURES 21-6 TO 21-11).

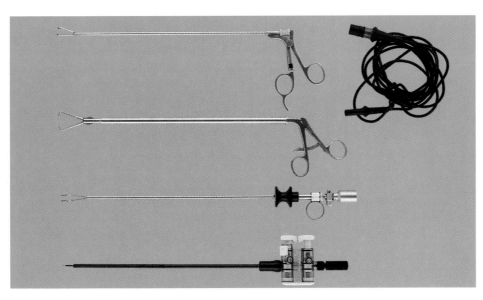

21-1 *Left, top to bottom,* 1 spring-loaded claw grasper, 5 mm; 1 single-toothed tenaculum, 10 mm; 1 Kleppinger forceps, 5 mm, 33 mm length; 1 Nezhat Dorsey monopolar needle with suction cannula (shown with disposable trumpet valve). *Right top,* 1 Kleppinger bipolar cord, 10 foot.

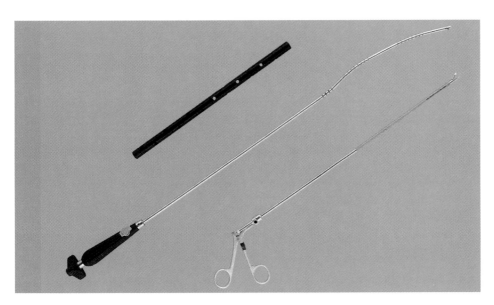

21-2 *Top to bottom,* 1 Endoflex protective cover; 1 Endoflex retractor, triangle, 5 mm, 80 mm length; 1 biopsy forceps, 5 mm.

21-3 *Top to bottom,* These are extra-long instruments; 1 Glassman (Hunter bowel grasper), 5 mm, 45 cm length; 1 Nezhat suction irrigator, 5 mm, 45 cm length; 1 Maryland dissector, monopolar, 5 mm.

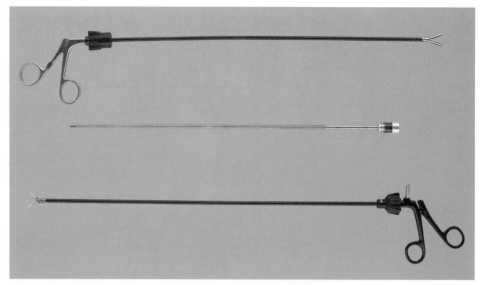

21-4 *Left to right,* Inlet fascial closure set: 3 incision-closure plugs (guides), 10, 12, and 15 mm; 1 needle point suture passer, 2.8 mm × 6 inch.

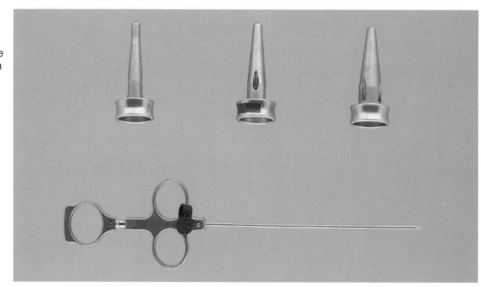

21-5 1 fiberoptic light cord, Wolf/Wolf ends for 5 and 10 mm laparoscope.

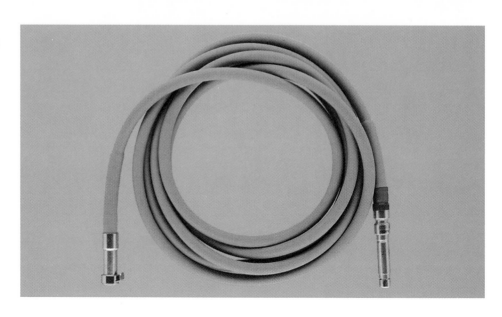

USED ON STANDARD AND LOW ANTERIOR COLON RESECTIONS (FIGURES 21-6 TO 21-11).

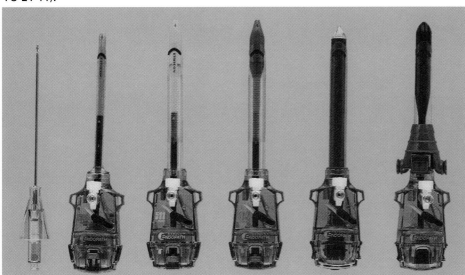

21-6 *Left to right,* 1 Verres needle, disposable; 3 dilating-tipped trocars, disposable, 5 mm, $^{10}/_{11}$ mm, 12 mm; 1 optical trocar, disposable, 10 mm; 1 blunt-tipped trocar (Hasson type), disposable, 10 mm.

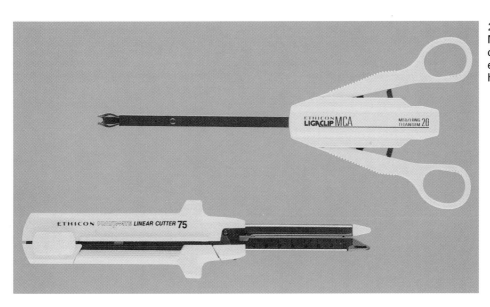

21-7 *Top to bottom,* Medium/large ligating and dividing ligaclip applier; linear cutter with reloadable head.

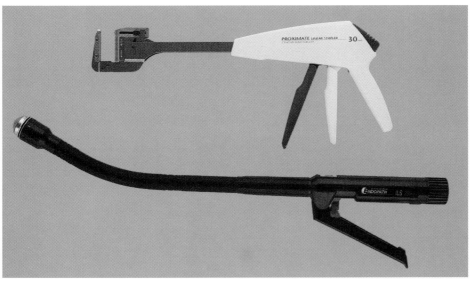

21-8 *Top to bottom,* Linear stapler, 30 mm; endoscopic circular stapler.

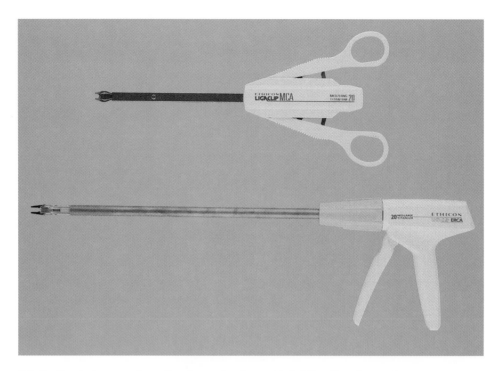

21-9 *Top to bottom,* 2 medium/large ligating and dividing ligaclip appliers.

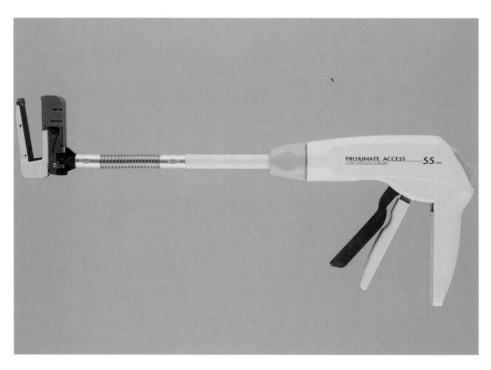

21-10 Linear stapler, 55 mm.

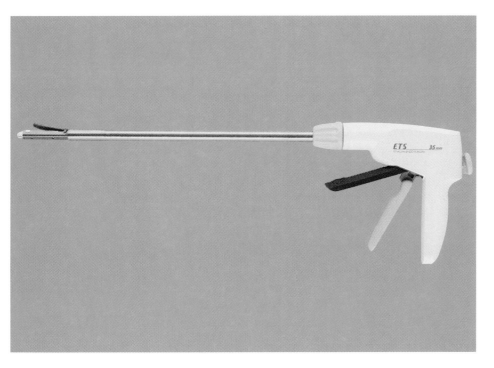

21-11 Endolinear cutter/stapler with reload unit.

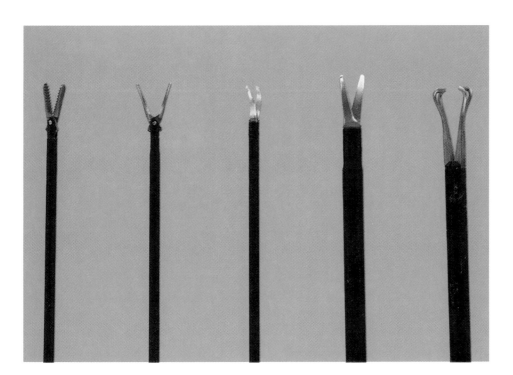

21-12 *Left to right,* Disposable instrument tips: grasping forceps, 5 mm; dissecting forceps, 5mm; Metzenbaum scissors, 5 mm; Metzenbaum scissors, 10 mm; and Babcock forceps, 10 mm.

LAPAROSCOPIC BOWEL RESECTION

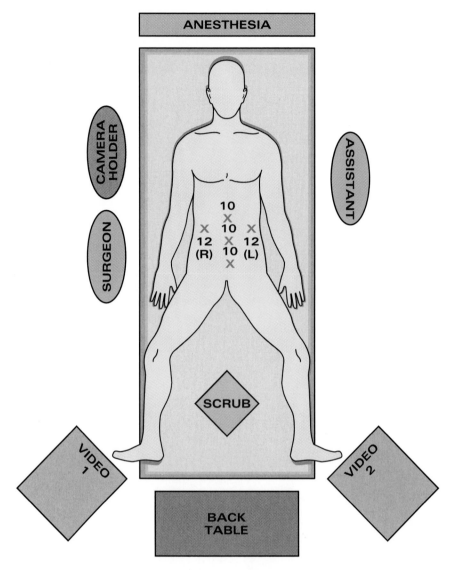

REVERSE FOR RIGHT SIDE
PATIENT IN LOW ALLEN STIRRUPS

21-13 Bowel resection.

LAPAROSCOPIC APPENDECTOMY

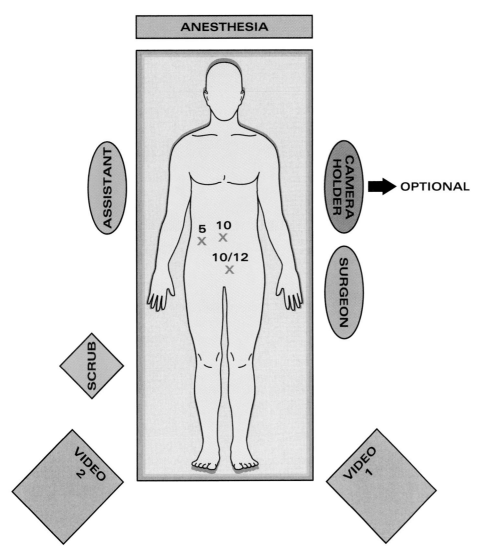

21-14 Appendectomy.

LAPAROSCOPIC HERNIA REPAIR (RIGHT SIDE)

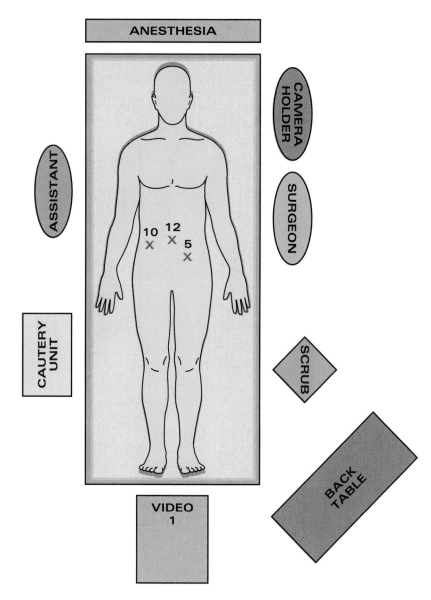

21-15 Hernia.

22

Thoracoscopy Instruments

ADD LAPAROSCOPIC ADVANCED SET, LAPAROSCOPE, LIGHT CORD, AND MINOR INSTRUMENT SET

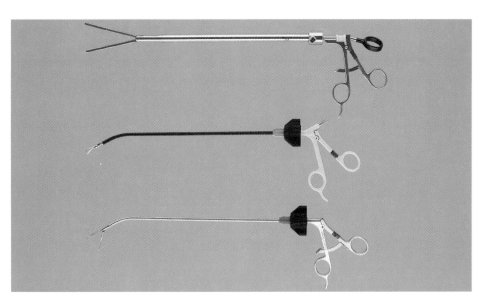

22-1 *Top to bottom,* 1 articulating lung grasper, 10 mm; 1 roticulating Metzenbaum scissors, 5 mm × 33 cm, angled shaft; 1 roticulating Babcock forceps, 5 mm × 33 cm, angled shaft.

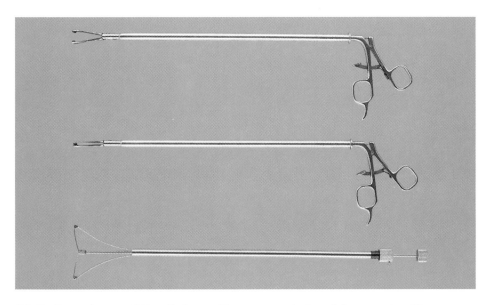

22-2 *Top to bottom,* 2 Duvall clamps 10mm, opened, closed; fan retractor, 10 mm (two parts).

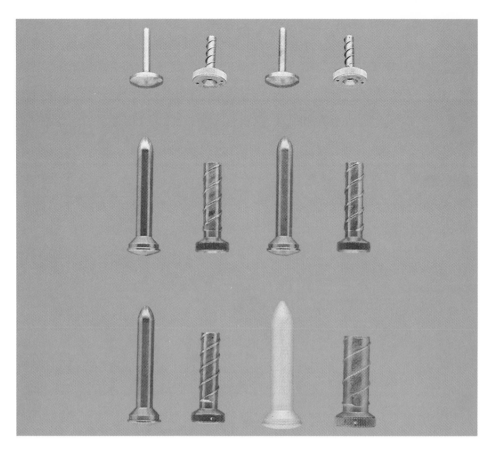

22-3 *Top*, 2 5 mm thoracoports, 1 blunt obturator, 1 cannula. *Middle*, 2 10 mm thora-coports, 1 blunt obturator, 1 cannula. *Bottom*, 1 12 mm and 1 15 mm thoracoport, 1 blunt obturator, 1 cannula.

THORACOSCOPY (LEFT)

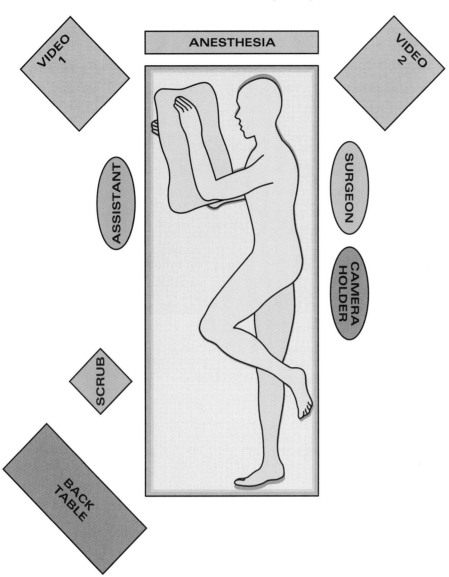

22-4 Thoracoscopy.

Vascular Instruments

ADD LAPAROSCOPIC ADVANCED SET, LAPAROSCOPE, LIGHT CORD, AND MINOR INSTRUMENT SET

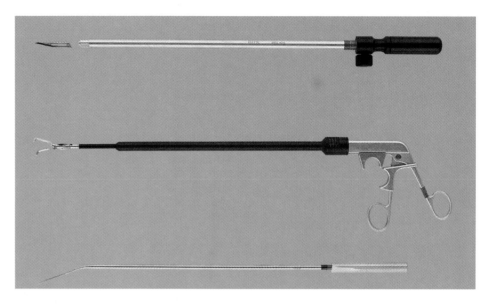

23-1 *Top to bottom,* 1 retracting knife handle with disposable (No. 11) blade, 10 mm; 1 Meeker right-angle forceps, 10 mm; 1 Penfield dissector, 5 mm, angled tip.

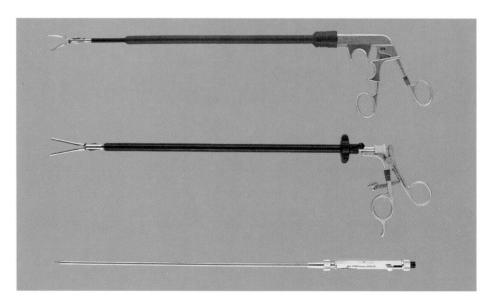

23-2 *Top to bottom,* 1 DeBakey forceps, 10 mm, curved tip, roticulating shaft; 1 Glassman forceps, 10 mm, ratcheted, roticulating shaft; 1 Berci retracting knife, 5 mm, with reusable blade.

Hysteroscopic Operative Instruments

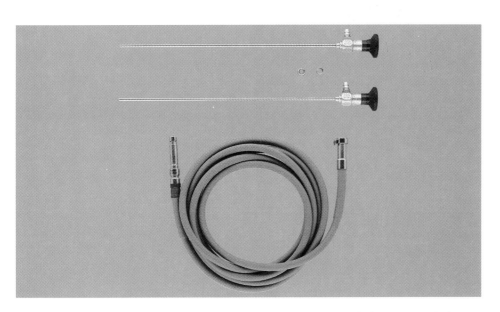

24-1 *Top to bottom,* Hysteroscopic operative set: 2 hysteroscopic lens, 4 mm; 0 degree, 30 degrees; 2 sealing caps and fiberoptic cord.

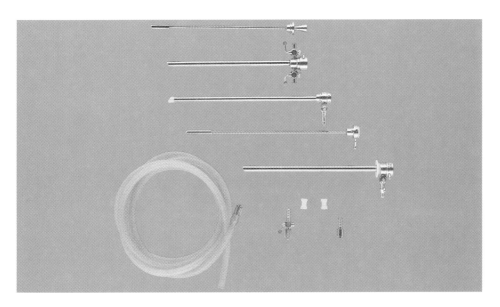

24-2 *Top to bottom, right,* For continous-flow operative hysteroscopy: 1 obturator, 21 Fr; 1 operative sheath, 21 Fr. For continous-flow resecting hysteroscopy: 1 inner sheath, 26 Fr; 1 obturator, 26 Fr; 1 outer sheath, 26 Fr. *Left bottom,* Outflow tubing with Luer-Lok connector on one end, 17 inches. *Right bottom, left to right,* 1 water connector with stop-cock; 2 gray nipples; 1 male Luer-Lok connector.

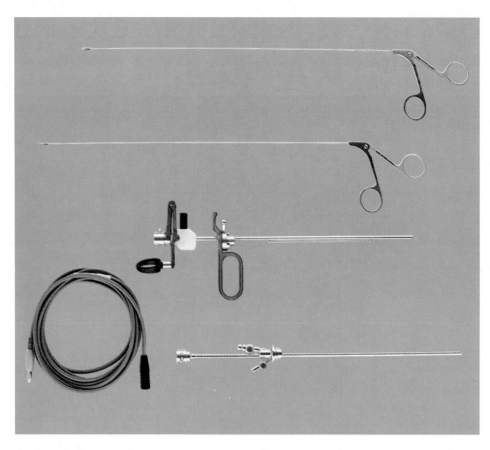

24-3 *Left bottom,* Monopolar cord, pin type. *Top to bottom,* For continous-flow operative hysteroscopy: 1 semirigid scissors, 7 Fr, 2.33 mm; 1 semirigid grasper, 7 Fr, 2.33 mm.
For continous-flow resecting hysteroscopy: 1 resecting working element. For continous-
flow operative hysteroscopy (used with the operative sheath, 21 Fr): 1 continous-flow
bridge with instrument channel.

25

Laparoscopic Tubal Ligation Set

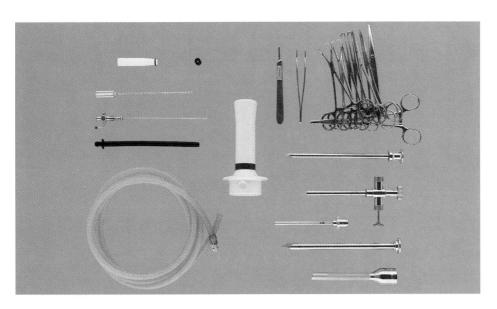

25-1 *Left, top to bottom,* 1 Fallopian ring pusher (with black ring); 1 black nipple; 1 Verres needle, medium; 1 Verres needle, stylet, medium; 1 reducer cannula, 5 mm, black; 1 insufflation tubing with Luer-Lok on one end. *Middle,* 1 light handle. *Right, top,* 1 Bard Parker knife handle, No. 3; 1 Adson tissue forceps with teeth (1 × 2); 2 Backhaus towel clips, large; 2 Allis tissue forceps; 2 Crile hemostatic forceps, curved; 1 Mayo dissecting scissors, straight; 1 Crile Wood needle holder, 7 inch. *Lower right, top to bottom,* 1 8 mm trocar and 1 trumpet-valve cannula (for Fallopian ring applier); 1 Applied cannula, 5 mm; 1 Applied trochar, 10/11mm; 1 Applied cannula, 10/11mm.

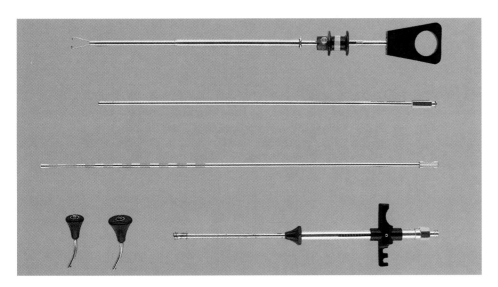

25-2 *Top to bottom,* 1 Fallopian ring applier, 7 mm; 1 suction or irrigation cannula; 1 manipulation probe; 1 Cohen cannula with two black tips.

HYSTEROSCOPIC PROCEDURES

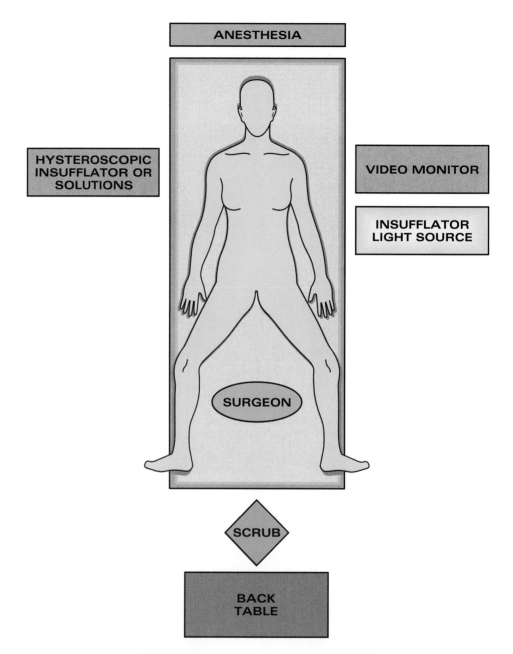

PATIENT IN LOW ALLEN STIRRUPS

25-3 Hysteroscopic procedures.

LAPAROSCOPIC TUBAL LIGATION

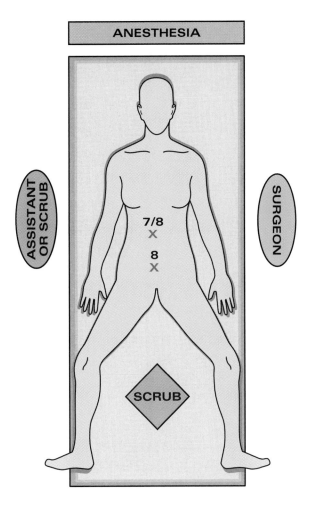

PATIENT IN LOW ALLEN STIRRUPS

25-4 Tubal ligation.

LAPAROSCOPIC GYNECOLOGIC PROCEDURES

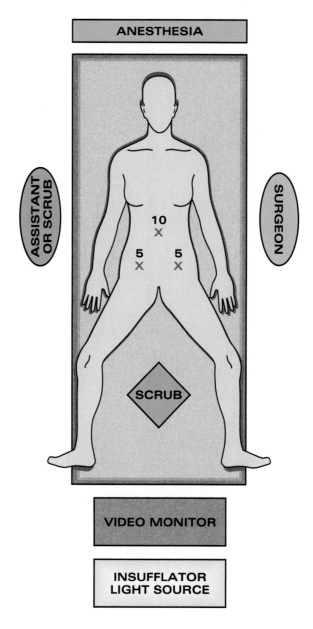

PATIENT IN LOW ALLEN STIRRUPS

25-5 Gynecologic procedures.

26

Laser Laparoscope

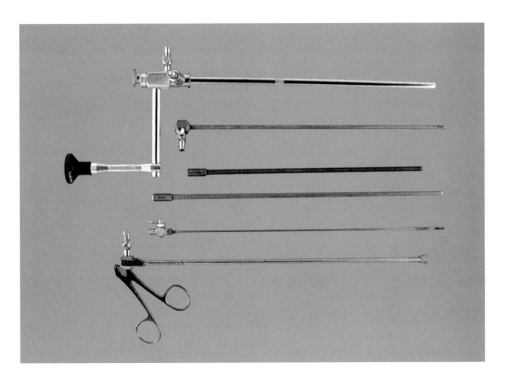

26-1 *Top to bottom,* 1 laser SL telescope; 1 aspirating/lavage outer cannula; 2 laser probes with calibration; 1 aspirating/lavage inner cannula; 1 irrigating/grasping forceps with offset handle.

27

Sigmoidoscopy Set

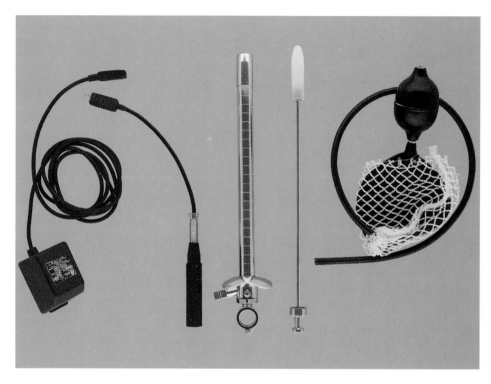

27-1 *Left to right,* 1 transformer cord; 1 light handle; 1 sigmoidoscope; 1 obturator; 1 colonic insufflator.

28

Paranasal Sinuses and Anterior Base of the Skull Instruments

ADDITIONAL EQUIPMENT: LIGHT SOURCE AND NASAL PAN
For irrigation: add cysto tubing, bag of normal saline and suction tubing.

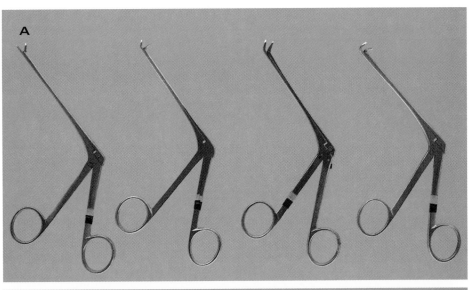

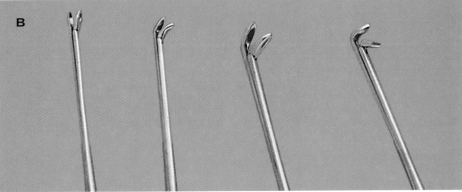

28-1 A, *Left to right,* Pediatric and small Weil-Blakesley ethmoid forceps: 1 pediatric straight, 1 pediatric 45 degree, 1 45 degree small, and 1 90 degree small. **B**, *Left to right,* Pediatric and small Weil-Blakesley ethmoid forceps, tips: 1 pediatric straight, 1 pediatric 45 degree, 1 45 degree small, and 1 90 degree small.

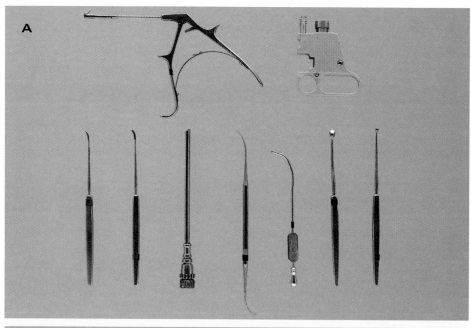

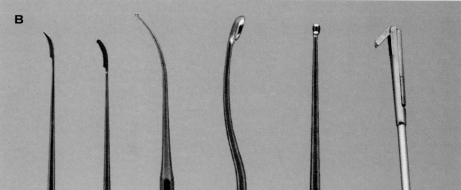

28-2 A, *Top, left to right,* 1 Stammberger antrum punch (backbiter); 1 axial suction/irrigation handle. *Bottom, left to right,* 2 sickle knives, sharp, blunt; 1 sheath for 0 and 25 degrees, 4 mm lens; 1 maxillary sinus seeker; 1 von Eicken antrum wash tube, 11 Fr; 2 sinus curettes, sizes 2 and 1. **B,** *Left to right,* Tips: 2 sickle knives, sharp, blunt; 1 maxillary sinus seeker; 2 sinus curettes, sizes 2 and 1; and 1 Stammberger antrum punch (backbiter).

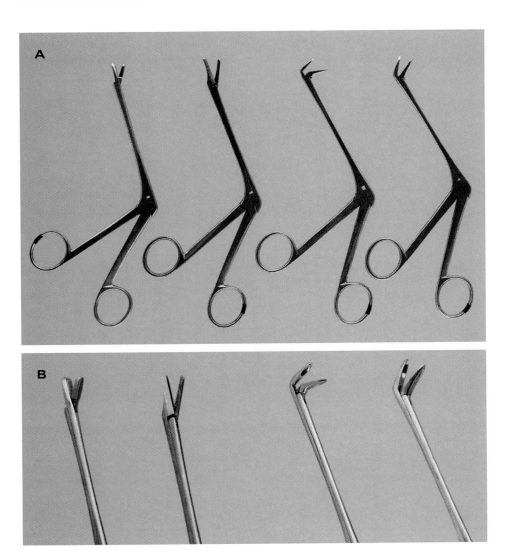

28-3 A, *Left to right,* Grünwald heuke nasal forceps, size 2: 1 straight, cutting; 1 Struycken nasal cutting forceps, size 2; 1 90 degree upward bent; and 1 upward bent. **B,** *Left to right,* Grünwald heuke nasal forceps, size 2, tips: 1 straight, cutting; 1 Struycken nasal cutting forceps, size 2; 1 90 degree upward bent; and 1 upward bent.

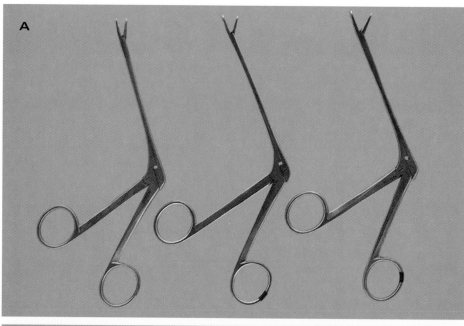

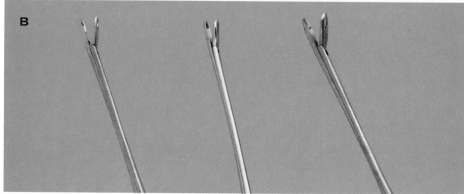

28-4 **A,** *Left to right,* Weil-Blakesley ethmoid forceps: 1 straight, size 0; 1 straight, size 1; and 1 straight, size 2. **B,** *Left to right,* Weil-Blakesley ethmoid forceps, tips: 1 straight, size 0; 1 straight, size 1; and 1 straight, size 2.

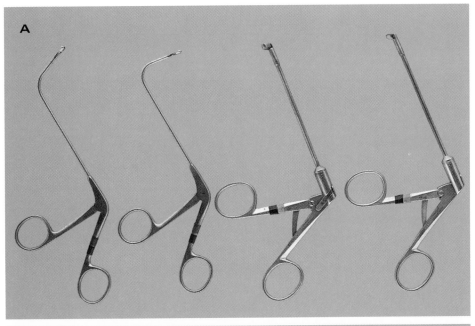

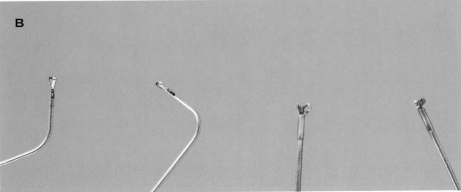

28-5 **A**, *Left to right,* 1 Kuhn-Bolger Giraffe forceps 90 degree (frontal sinus punch); 1 Kuhn-Bolger Giraffe forceps 110 degree (frontal sinus punch); 2 Stammberger antrum punches, left, right. **B**, *Left to right,* tips: 1 Kuhn-Bolger Giraffe forceps 90 degree; 1 Kuhn-Bolger Giraffe forceps 110 degree; and 2 Stammberger antrum punches, left, right.

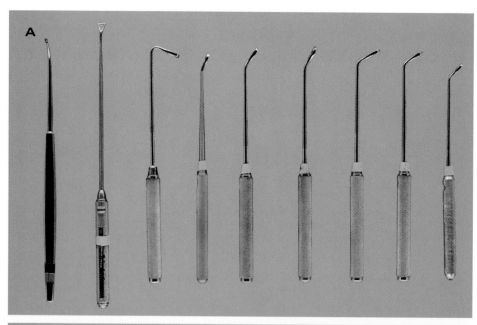

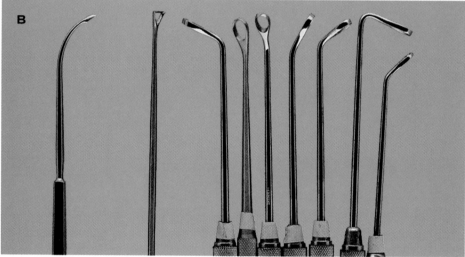

28-6 **A,** *Left to right,* 1 frontal sinus curette 90 degree; 1 Coakley antrum curette, straight with triangle tip; variety of Coakley antrum curettes with various angles and sizes 1-6. **B,** *Left to right,* Tips: frontal sinus curette and a variety of Coakley antrum currettes with various angles and sizes 1-6.

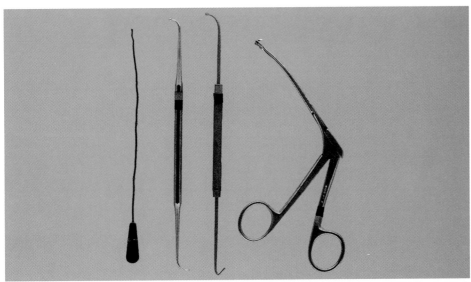

28-7 *Left to right,* 1 beaded measuring probe; 1 maxillary sinus ostium seeker; 1 frontal ostium seeker; 1 Ostrom Terrier ostium forceps, retrograde.

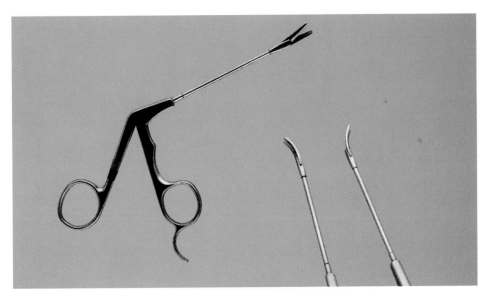

28-8 *Left to right,* 1 small nasal scissors, straight. Tips: small nasal scissors, curved left, curved right.

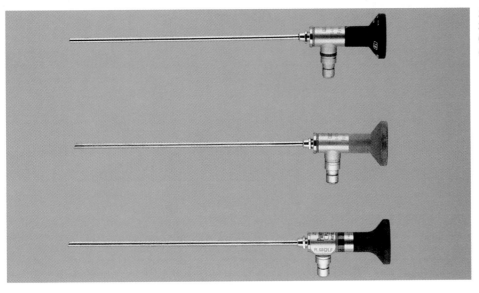

28-9 *Top to bottom,* 3 telescope lens 4 mm: 0 degree, 25 degree, 70 degree.

Small Joint Arthroscope

ADD 1 BARD PARKER KNIFE HANDLE, NO. 3; ADSON TISSUE FORCEPS WITH TEETH (1 × 2); 1 STRAIGHT MAYO DISSECTING SCISSORS; 1 HALSTEAD MOSQUITO HEMOSTATIC FORCEPS, CURVED; AND 1 WEBSTER NEEDLE HOLDER

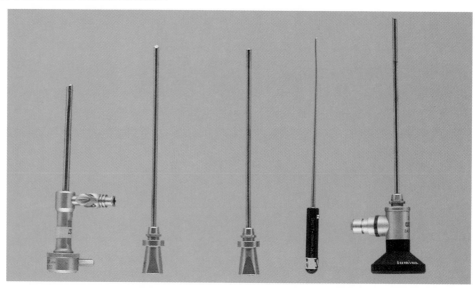

29-1 *Left to right,* 1 trocar sleeve, 2.7 mm; 1 pyramidal trocar; 1 blunt obturator; 1 probe; 1 telescope lens, 25 degree.

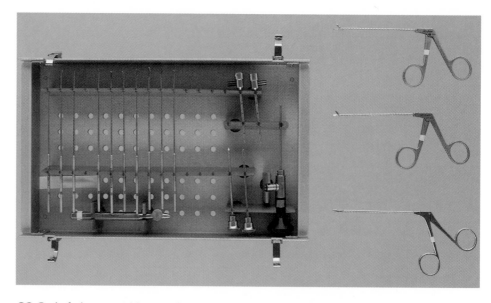

29-2 *Left, in case,* 1 blunt probe; 1 hook probe; 1 straight rasp; 1 angled-down rasp; 1 angled-up rasp; 1 lateral-release knife; 1 retrograde knife; 1 serrated banana knife; 1 meniscectomy knife, right; 1 meniscectomy knife, left; 1 handle. *Right, top,* 1 blunt obturator; 1 pyramidal trocar; *right, bottom,* 2 trocar sleeves and telescope lens, 30 degree. *Right, top to bottom, not in case,* 1 cup forceps; 1 scissors; 1 grasper.

Carpal Tunnel Instruments

ADD 1 BARD PARKER KNIFE HANDLE, NO. 3; 1 MAYO DISSECTING SCISSORS, STRAIGHT; 1 ADSON TISSUE FORCEPS WITH TEETH (1 × 2); AND 1 CRILE WOOD NEEDLE HOLDER.

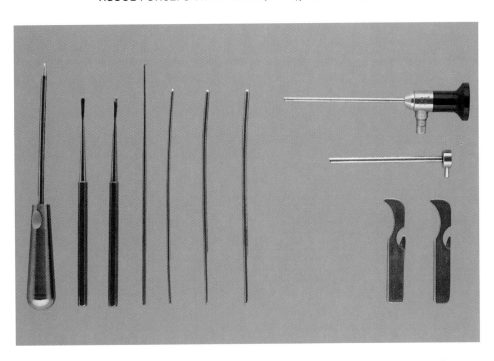

30-1 *Left to right,* 1 ridged obturator; 1 straight blunt dissector; 1 curved blunt dissector; 1 right-angle probe; 3 Hegar dilators (3, 4, and 5). *Top, right,* 1 carpal tunnel video endoscope, 30 degree; 1 slotted cannula; 2 gold handles for disposable carpal tunnel blades.

Knee Arthroscopic Instrument Set

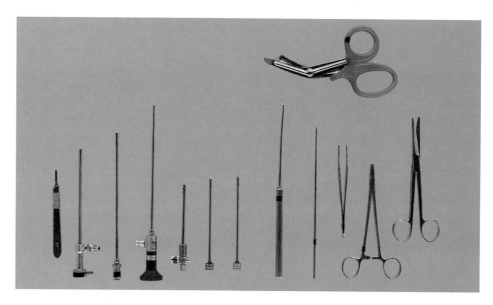

31-1 *Top, right,* Large bandage scissors. *Bottom, left to right,* 1 Bard Parker knife handle, No. 3; 1 self-locking trocar sleeve, 4 mm; 1 blunt obturator, 4 mm; 1 Lumina telescope, 25 degree, 4 mm; 1 egress cannula, 4.5 mm; 1 pyramidal trocar, 3.7 mm; 1 conical obturator, 3.7 mm; 2 probes; 1 Adson tissue forceps with teeth (1 × 2); 1 Crile Wood needle holder, 6 inch; 1 Mayo dissecting scissors, straight.

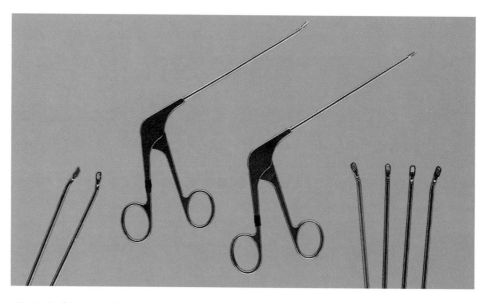

31-2 *Left to right,* Tips: 2 Acufex Duckbill biters, right, left; 1 Acufex Duckbill biter, upbite; 1 Acufex Duckbill biter, straight bite. Tips: 4 Acufex Ducklings bill biters, right, upbite, straight, left.

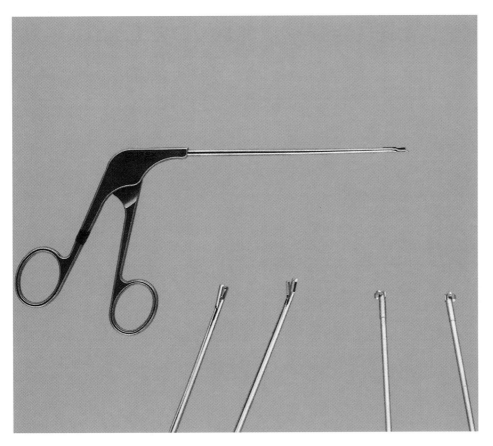

31-3 *Left to right,* 1 grasper. Tips: 2 Acufex upbiting linear punches, 1.3 mm, 1.5 mm; 2 Acufex baskets, 90 degree, 2.2 mm, left and right.

32

Stryker Battery Power Drill

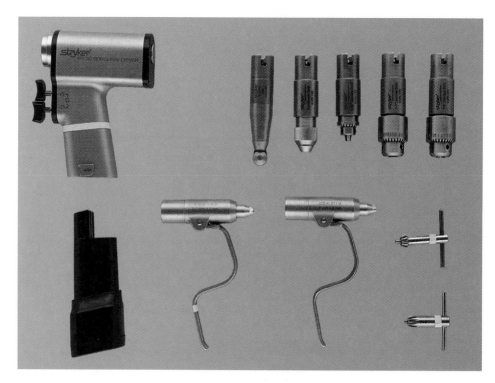

32-1 *Left, top to bottom,* 1 Stryker drill; 1 power pack. *Right top, left to right,* 1 sagittal saw attachment; 1 Synthes chuck; 1 Jacob $^5/_{32}$ chuck; 2 Jacob $^1/_4$ chucks. *Right bottom, left to right,* 2 pin collets, 3 mm (1.2), 7 mm (1.8); 2 chuck keys.

33

Arthroscopic Anterior Cruciate Ligament Reconstruction with Patellar Tendon Bone Graft Instruments

ADD KNEE ARTHROSCOPIC INSTRUMENT SET, ARTHROSCOPIC WAND, AND ARTHROSCOPIC SHAVER

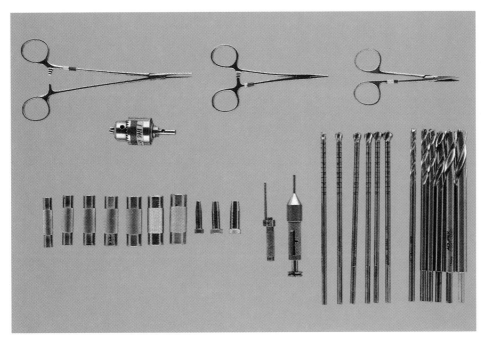

33-1 *Top, left to right,* 1 hemostatic tonsil forceps, straight; 1 Webster needle holder, 5 inch; 1 small sharp scissors. *Middle,* 1 Jacobs chuck. *Bottom, left to right,* 7 Acufex graft sizers, 6 mm to 12 mm; 3 Acufex isometric centering guides, 7-8 mm, 9-10 mm, 11 mm; 1 parallel drill guide, 5 mm; 1 isometric positioner; 6 acorn cannulated drill bits for femoral drilling; 6 Acufex cannulated drill bits for tibial drilling.

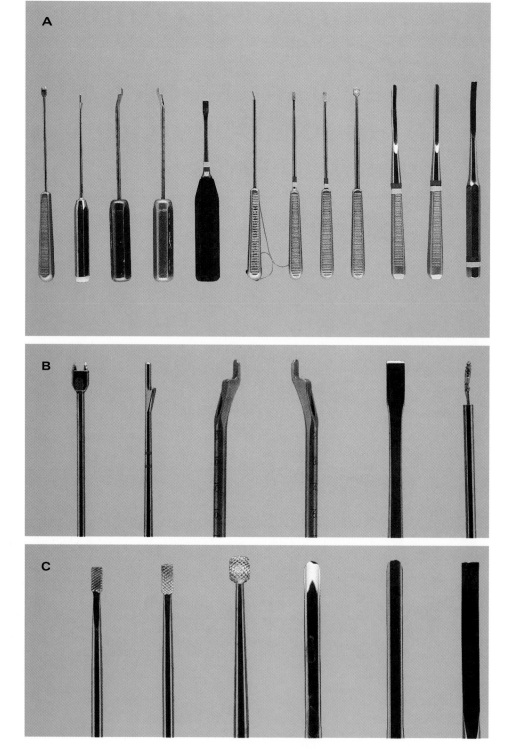

33-2 A, *Left to right,* 1 Arthrex graft pusher; 1 Arthrex femoral tunnel notcher; 1 Arthrex over the top femoral positioning drill guide, 6 mm; 1 Arthrex over the top femoral positioning drill guide, 7 mm; 1 osteotome, thin $^1/_4$ inch; 1 Isotac screwdriver with suture and isotac in place; 3 chamfering rasps, convex, concave, half round; 2 gouges, $^1/_4$ inch: straight, curved; 1 osteotome, $^1/_4$ inch, curved. **B,** *Left to right,* 5 Arthrex tips: graft pusher; femoral tunnel notcher; over the top femoral positioning drill guide, 6 mm; over the top femoral positioning drill guide, 7 mm; osteotome $^1/_4$ inch, thin; and Isotac screwdriver with suture and isotac in place. **C,** *Left to right,* 3 rasp tips: convex, concave, and half round; 2 gouges $^1/_4$ inch, tips: straight, curved; 1 osteotome $^1/_4$ inch, curved.

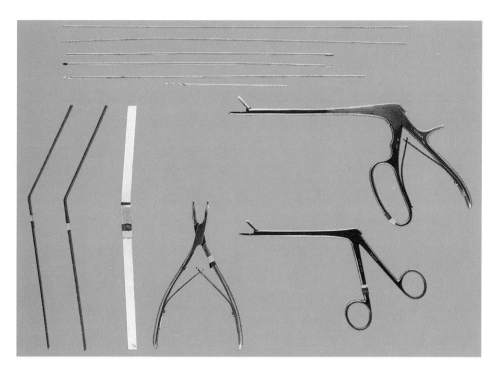

33-3 *Top to bottom,* 2 Hyperflex guide wires; 2 Beath passing pins; 1 drill bit, $^1/_{16}$ inch. *Bottom, left to right,* 3 templates, 8, 9, 10, side view, front view; 1 Beyer rongeur curved; 1 Ferris-Smith rongeur, cup jaw (Martin); 1 Pituitary rongeur.

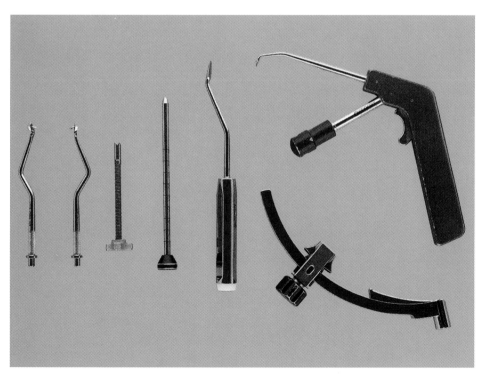

33-4 *Left to right,* 2 tibial aiming hooks, right, left, for Arthrex tibial guide; 1 K wire sleeve for Concept precise tibial aiming guide; 1 K wire sleeve for Arthrex tibial aiming guide; 1 notchplasty gouge. *Right, top to bottom,* 1 Concept precise tibial aiming guide; 1 Arthrex tibial aiming guide.

34

Shoulder Arthroscopic Instruments

ADD KNEE ARTHROSCOPIC INSTRUMENT SET

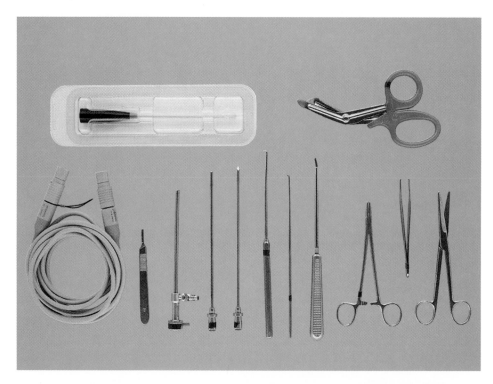

34-1 *Top, left to right,* 1 arthroscopic wand (bipolar coagulator) in sterile package; 1 heavy scissors. *Bottom, left to right,* Bipolar cord; 1 Bard Parker knife handle, No. 3; 1 telescope sheath, 5 mm; 2 obturators, dull, sharp, 5 mm; 2 nerve hooks, large, small; 1 convex rasp; 1 Crile Wood needle holder, 6 inch; 1 Adson tissue forceps with teeth (1 × 2); 1 Mayo dissecting scissors, straight.

VAGINAL AND RECTAL SURGERY

35

Vaginal Set

35-1 *Left to right,* 2 Bard Parker knife handles, No. 4; 1 Bard Parker knife handle, No. 4, long; 1 Mayo dissecting scissors, straight; 1 Metzenbaum scissors, 7 inch; 1 Mayo dissecting scissors, curved; 1 Mayo dissecting scissors, long, curved; 2 Ferris-Smith tissue forceps; 2 Russian tissue forceps; 1 tissue forceps without teeth, long.

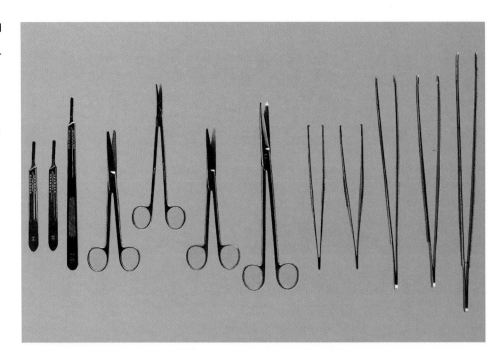

35-2 *Top to bottom,* 1 uterine sound; 1 Yankauer suction tube with tip. *Left to right,* 4 paper drape clips; 2 Backhaus towel clips; 8 Crile hemostatic forceps, 6½ inch; 4 Halstead hemostatic forceps; 12 Allis tissue forceps; 6 Allis-Adair tissue forceps; 4 tonsil hemostatic forceps; 2 Heaney needle holders; 2 Crile Wood needle holders, 8 inch; 2 Heaney hysterectomy forceps; 2 Ballentine Heaney hysterectomy forceps; 2 Ochsner hemostatic forceps, 8 inch; 2 Allis tissue forceps, long; 2 Babcock tissue forceps, medium; 2 Schroeder uterine tenaculum forceps, single tooth; 1 Skene uterine vulsellum forceps, double tooth, straight; 2 Foerster sponge forceps.

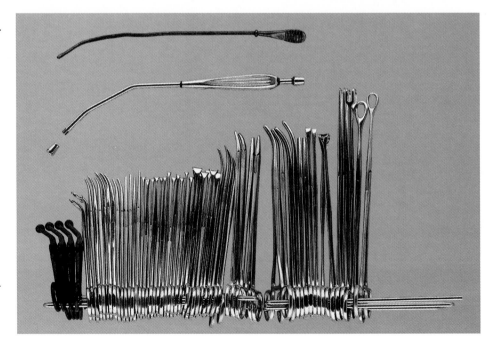

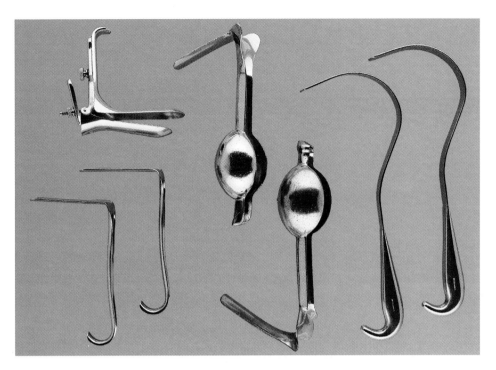

35-3 *Top, left to right,* 1 Graves vaginal speculum; 1 Auvard weighted vaginal speculum, medium lip. *Bottom, left to right,* 2 Heaney retractors; 1 Auvard weighted vaginal speculum, long lip; 2 Deaver retractors, narrow.

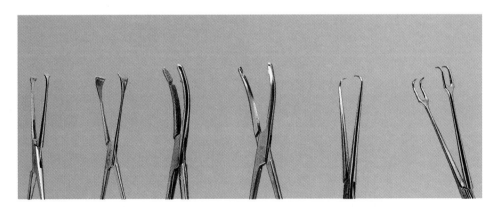

35-4 *Left to right,* Tips: 1 Allis tissue forceps; 1 Allis-Adair tissue forceps; 1 Heaney hysterectomy forceps; 1 Ballentine Heaney hysterectomy forceps; 1 Schroeder uterine tenaculum forceps, single tooth; 1 Skene uterine vulsellum forceps, double tooth, straight.

36

Dilatation and Curettage Set

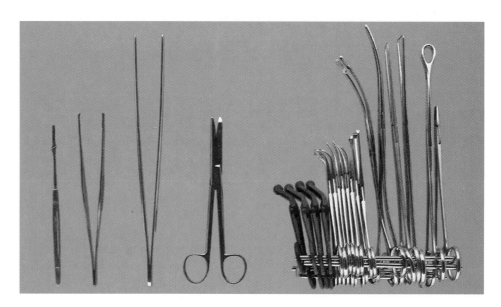

36-1 *Left to right,* 1 Bard Parker knife handle, No. 7; 1 Ferris-Smith tissue forceps; 1 tissue forceps without teeth, long; 1 Mayo dissecting scissors, curved; 4 paper drape clips; 2 Backhaus towel forceps; 4 Crile hemostatic forceps, 5½ inch; 2 Allis tissue forceps; 1 Randall stone forceps, ¼ curve; 1 thumb dressing forceps; 2 Schroeder uterine tenaculum forceps, single tooth; 1 Foerster sponge forceps; 1 Crile Wood needle holder, 7 inch.

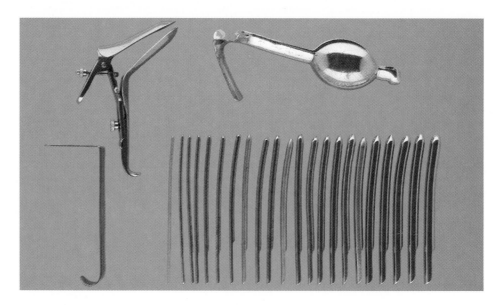

36-2 *Top, left to right,* 1 Graves vaginal speculum; 1 Auvard weighted vaginal speculum, medium lip. *Bottom, left to right,* 1 Heaney retractor; 1 set of Hegar dilators, sizes 3 to 13½ (including half sizes).

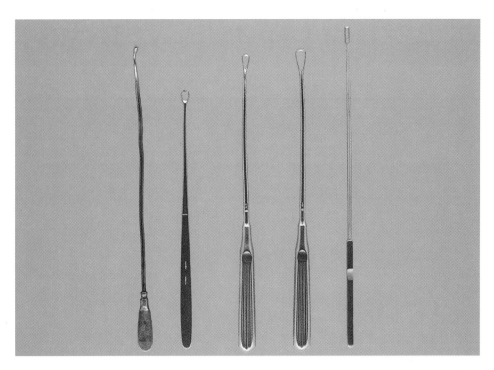

36-3 *Left to right,* 1 Sims uterine sound; 1 Heaney uterine curette, sharp, serrated tip; 1 Thomas uterine curette semirigid, dull, small; 1 Sims uterine curette semirigid, sharp, medium; 1 Kevorkian curette.

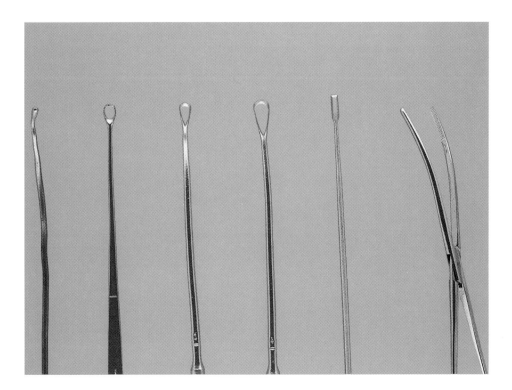

36-4 *Left to right,* Tips: 1 Sims uterine sound; 1 Heaney uterine curette, sharp, serrated tip; 1 Thomas uterine curette, semirigid, dull, small; 1 Sims uterine curette, semirigid, sharp, medium; 1 Kevorkian curette; thumb dressing forceps.

37

Rectal and Pilonidal Cyst Set

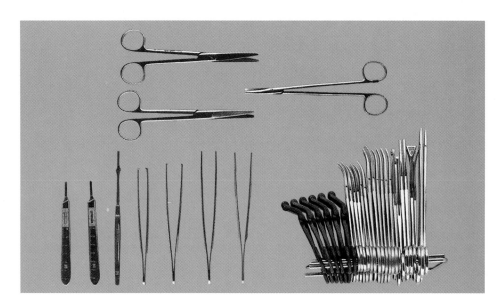

37-1 *Top, left to right,* 2 Mayo dissecting scissors, straight; 1 Metzenbaum scissors, 7 inch. *Bottom, left to right,* 2 Bard Parker knife handles, No. 3; 1 Bard Parker knife handle, No. 7; 2 thumb tissue forceps with teeth (1 × 2); 2 DeBakey Autraugrip tissue forceps, short; 6 paper drape clips; 6 Crile hemostatic forceps, 5½ inch; 6 Crile hemostatic forceps, 6½ inch; 2 Allis tissue forceps; 2 Ochsner hemostatic forceps, short; 2 Pennington hemostatic forceps; 2 Crile Wood needle holders, 7 inch.

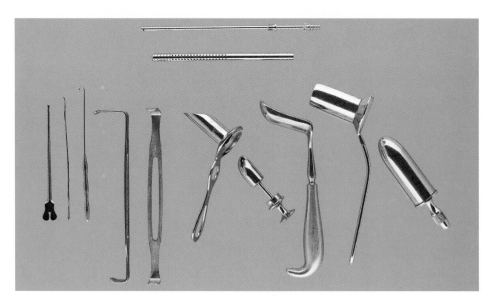

37-2 *Top,* 1 Poole abdominal suction tube and shield. *Bottom, left to right,* 1 grooved director; 1 probe dilator; 1 Rosser crypt hook; 2 Army Navy retractors, side view, front view; 1 Hirschmann anoscope (2 parts); 1 Hill-Ferguson rectal retractor; 1 anoscope, extra large.

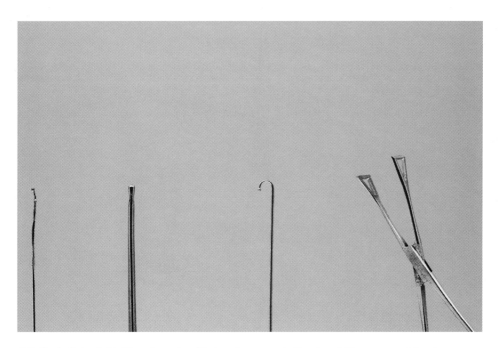

37-3 *Left to right,* Tips: 1 probe dilator; 1 grooved director; 1 Rosser crypt hook; 1 Pennington hemostatic forceps.

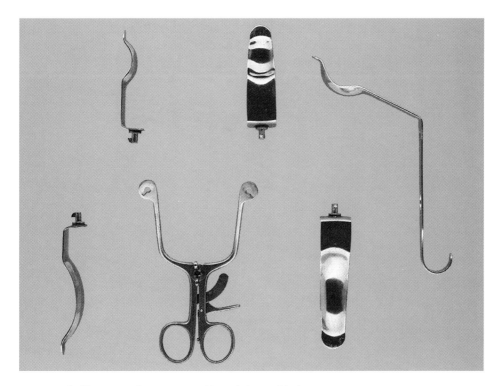

37-4 1 Sullivan rectal retractor, self-retaining, 5 blades.

Unit Six

NEUROSURGERY

Neuro Soft Tissue Set

38-1 *Top to bottom, left to right,* 2 Bard Parker knife handles, No. 7; 2 Bard Parker knife handles, No. 3; 1 bipolar cautery forceps, dull, bayonet shaft; 1 Adson hypophyseal forceps, bayonet shaft; 1 Gerald tissue forceps, bayonet shaft; 1 thumb dressing forceps without teeth, bayonet shaft. *Bottom, left to right,* 2 Adson tissue forceps with teeth (1 × 2); 2 fine Gyne tissue forceps with teeth (1 × 2); 2 DeBakey Autraugrip tissue forceps, medium; 2 Gerald tissue forceps with teeth (1 × 2); 2 Cushing tissue forceps with teeth (1 × 2); 2 vital Cushing tissue forceps with teeth (1 × 2).

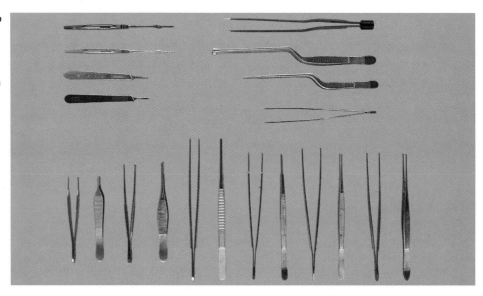

38-2 *Top to bottom, left to right,* 1 Mayo dissecting scissors, straight; 1 Metzenbaum scissors, 7 inch; 1 Metzenbaum scissors, 5 inch; 1 Strully scissors; 1 Stevens tenotomy scissors, straight. *Bottom, left to right,* 2 Rainey clip appliers; 3 paper drape clips; 2 ligaclip appliers, small/short; 4 Backhaus towel forceps; 6 Backhaus towel forceps, small; 6 Cairn hemostatic forceps; 6 Crile hemostatic forceps, curved; 2 Allis tissue forceps; 2 Ochsner tissue forceps; 2 ligaclip appliers, medium/medium; 1 Westphal hemostatic forceps; 1 Adson hemostatic forceps, fine tip; 2 DeBakey needle holders, 7 inch; 2 Webster needle holders, 6 inch; 2 Crile Wood needle holders, 7 inch.

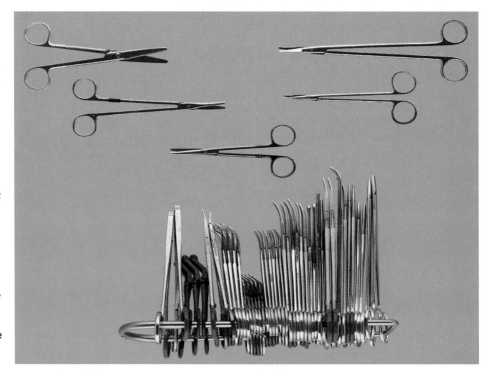

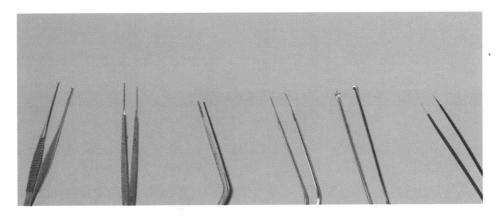

38-3 *Left to right,* Tips: fine Gyne tissue forceps with teeth (1 × 2); Gerald tissue forceps with teeth (1 × 2); thumb tissue forceps, bayonet shaft without teeth; Gerald tissue forceps without teeth, bayonet shaft; Adson hypophyseal forceps, bayonet shaft; bipolar cautery forceps, dull.

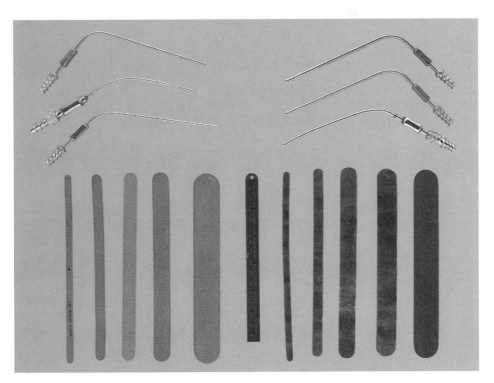

38-4 *Top left to right,* 6 Frazier suction tubes, sizes 6 to 12. *Bottom, left to right,* 5 silicone spatula retractors, 6, 9, 13, 16, and 22 mm; 1 metal ruler; 5 metal spatula retractors, various widths.

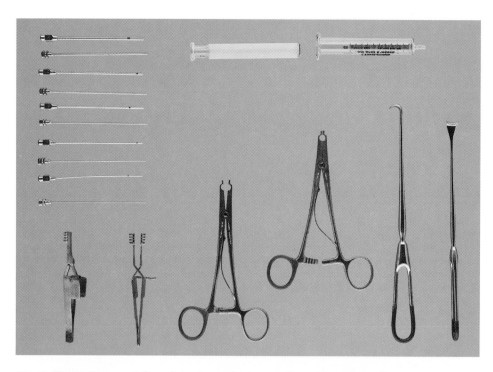

38-5 *Top to bottom, left to right,* 5 ventricular needles with stylets, 3½ inch, 12, 14, 16, 18, and 20 gauge; 1 10 ml glass-tipped syringe (2 parts). *Bottom, left to right,* 2 Heintz self-retaining retractors, small; 2 Rainey clip appliers, side view; 2 vein retractors, side view, front view.

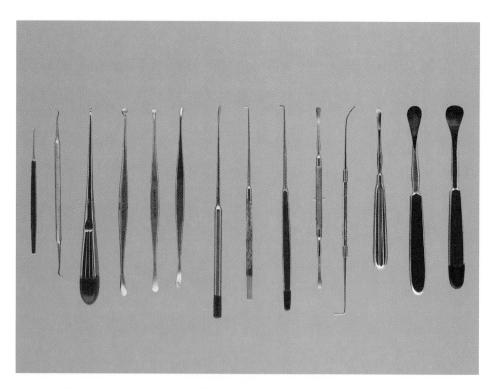

38-6 *Left to right,* 1 dura hook; 1 Woodson dura elevator; 1 Spratt curette, angled, 3-0; 3 Penfield dissectors, No. 1, 2, and 4; 1 probe, dull; 1 nerve hook, sharp; 1 nerve hook, dull, flat; 1 Freer elevator; 1 Kistner probe; 1 Love Adson elevator (joker); 2 Hoen periosteal elevators, narrow, wide.

39

Neuro Bone Pan Instruments

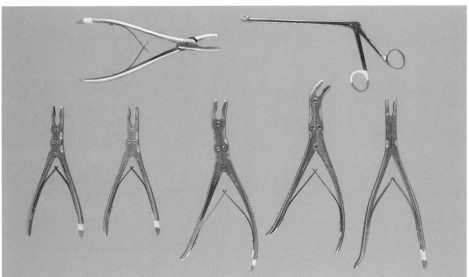

39-1 *Top left to right,* 1 Adson rongeur; 1 cup rongeur, 6mm. *Bottom, left to right,* 2 Ruskin double-action rongeurs, small straight, small curved; 2 Leksell rongeurs, side curved, curved; 1 Smith-Peterson laminectomy rongeur.

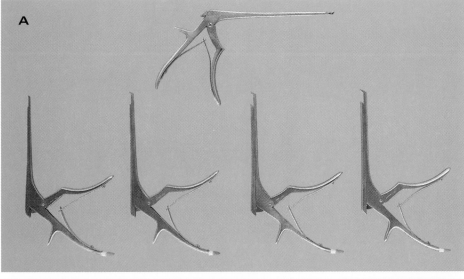

39-2 A, *Top,* 1 Kerrison rongeur, 45 degree, 1 mm. *Bottom, left to right,* 4 Kerrison rongeurs, 45 degree, 2, 3, 4, and 5 mm. **B**, *Left to right,* Tips: 5 Kerrison rongeurs, 45 degree, 1, 2, 3, 4, and 5 mm.

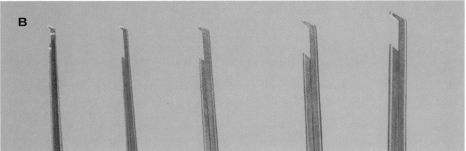

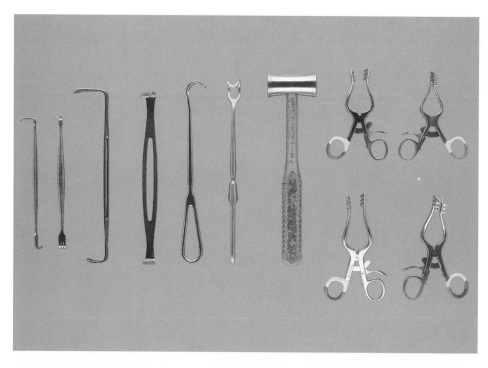

39-3 *Left to right,* 2 Senn retractors, side view, front view; 2 Army Navy retractors, side view, front view; 2 Green goiter retractors; 1 metal mallet. *Top to bottom, left to right,* 2 Weitlaner retractors, baby, angled; 2 Weitlaner retractors, small, angled.

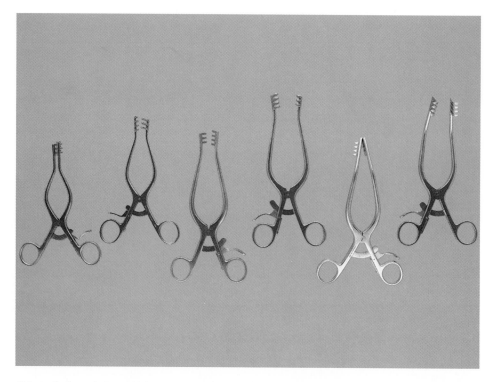

39-4 *Left to right,* 2 Weitlaner retractors, small; 2 Weitlaner retractors, medium; 2 Adson retractors, sharp, medium, angled.

Neuro Retractors

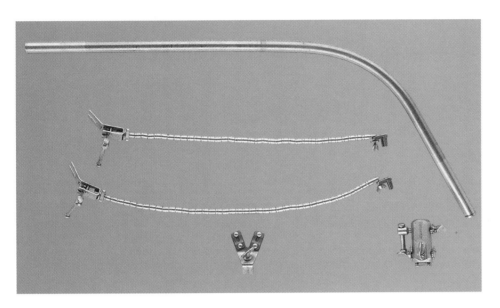

40-1 Leyla retractor, 1 fixation base for the 2 flexible arms, square block, table brace.

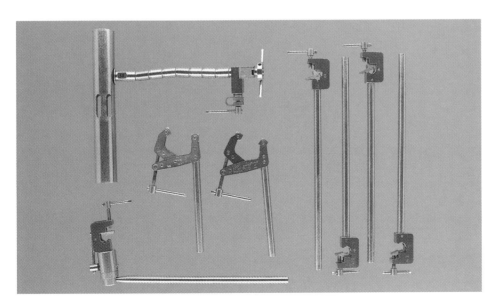

40-2 *Top to bottom, left to right,* Greenberg retractor: hand rest, flexible bar at clamp, 2 bars with clamps, 4 primary bars.

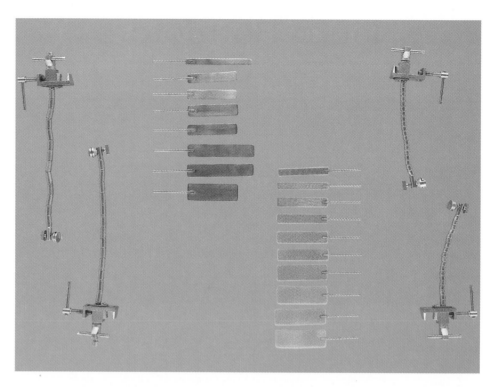

40-3 Greenberg retractor continued: 4 flexible retractor bars, long, short. *Middle, top to bottom,* 8 metal brain spatulas, various widths; 10 plastic-coated blades, various widths.

Rhoton Neuro Micro Instrument Set

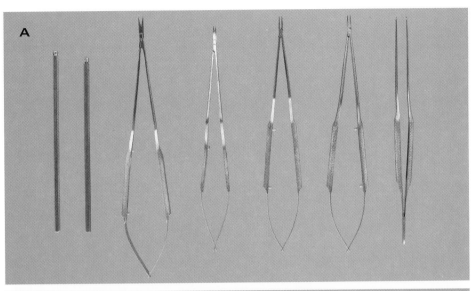

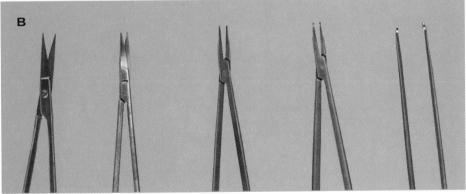

41-1 A, *Left to right,* 2 Beaver blade handles with insert, knurled; 1 microscissors, straight; 1 microscissors, curved; 1 micro-needle holder, straight; 1 micro-needle holder, curved; 1 micro-grasping forceps. **B,** *Left to right,* Tips: 2 microscissors, straight, curved; 2 micro-needle holders, straight, curved; 1 micro-grasping forceps.

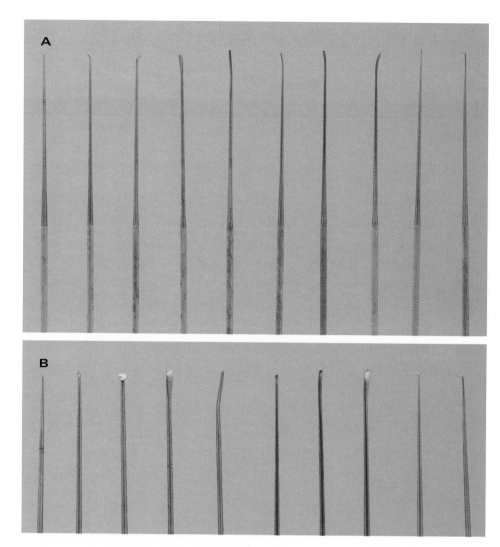

41-2 **A**, *Left to right,* 3 round microdissectors, 1, 2, and 3 mm; 2 general purpose microelevators, curved, angled; 3 spatula microdissectors, small, medium, large; 2 microhooks, 90 degree, semisharp, blunt; and, **B**, tips.

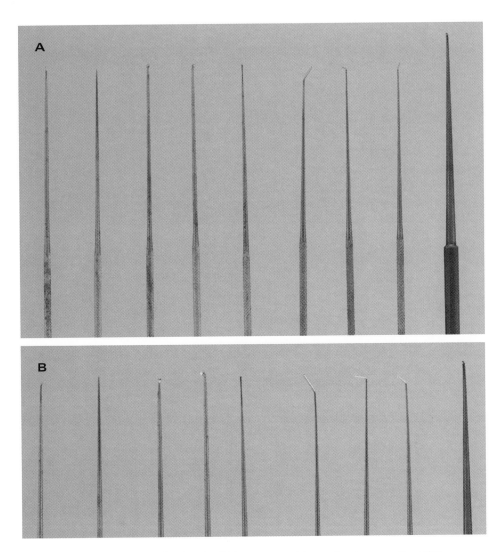

41-3 A, *Left to right,* 1 microhook, 45 degree, semisharp; 1 micro-needle point, straight; 2 microcurettes, straight, angled; 4 ball microdissectors: straight; 90 degree, 5 mm; 40 degree, 4 mm; 40 degree, 8 mm; 1 arachnoid microknife; and, **B,** tips.

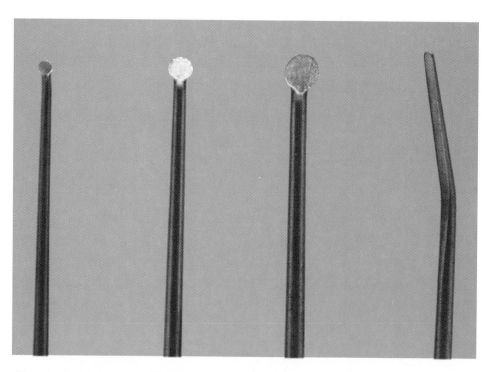

41-4 *Left to right,* Enlarged tips: 3 round microdissectors, 1, 2, and 3 mm; 1 general purpose microelevator, angled.

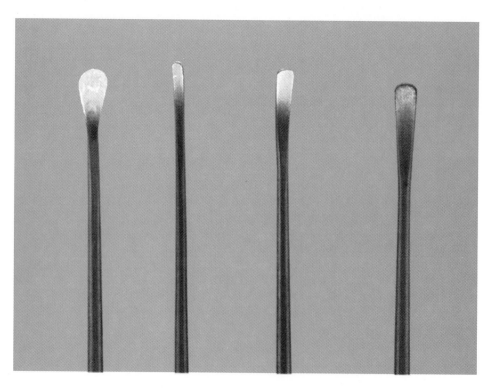

41-5 *Left to right,* Enlarged tips: 4 spatula microdissectors, large, small, medium, and medium straight.

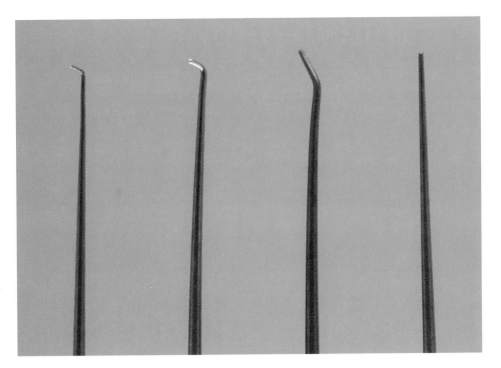

41-6 *Left to right,* Enlarged tips: 2 microhooks, 90 degree, semisharp, blunt; 1 general purpose microelevator, curved; 1 micro-needle point, straight.

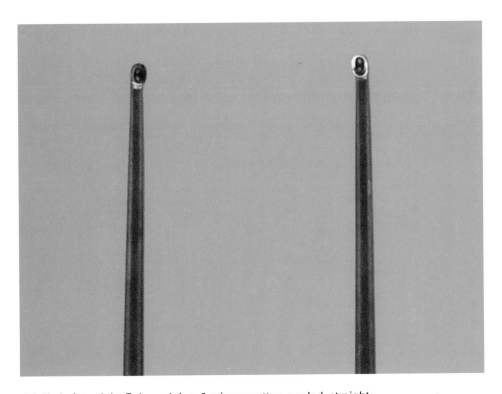

41-7 *Left to right,* Enlarged tips: 2 microcurettes, angled, straight.

42

Neuro Shunt Instruments

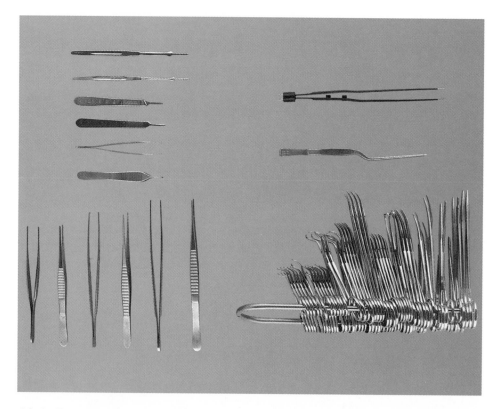

42-1 *Top to bottom, left to right,* 2 Bard Parker knife handles, No. 7; 2 Bard Parker knife handles, No. 3; 2 Adson tissue forceps with teeth; 1 bipolar cautery forceps; 1 thumb dressing forceps without teeth. *Bottom, left to right,* 2 DeBakey Autraugrip tissue forceps, short; 2 Cushing tissue forceps with teeth (1 × 2); 2 DeBakey Autraugrip tissue forceps, medium; 12 Backhaus towel forceps, small; 4 Backhaus towel forceps; 4 tonsil hemostatic forceps, short; 4 tonsil hemostatic forceps, long; 6 Halstead mosquito hemostatic forceps, curved; 2 Allis tissue forceps; 4 Crile hemostatic forceps, curved; 1 Iris scissors; 1 Stevens tenotomy scissors; 2 Metzenbaum scissors, 5 inch, 7 inch; 1 Mayo dissecting scissors, straight; 1 Webster needle holder, 4 1/2 inch; 1 Sarot needle holder; 1 Ryder needle holder; 2 Crile Wood needle holders, 7 inch.

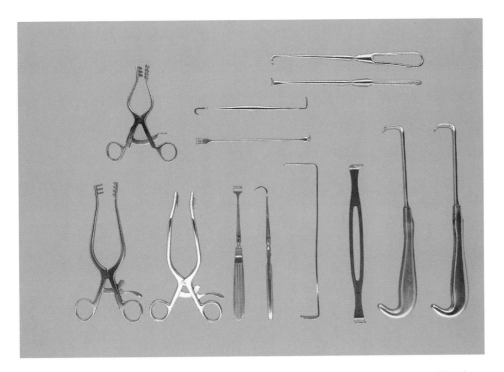

42-2 *Top, left to right,* 1 Weitlaner retractor, small, angled; 2 Senn retractors, side view, front view; 2 vein retractors. *Bottom, left to right,* 1 Weitlaner retractor, medium; 1 Adson retractor, angled; 2 Cushing vein and nerve retractor, front view, side view; 2 Army Navy retractors, side view, front view; 2 Richardson retractors, baby.

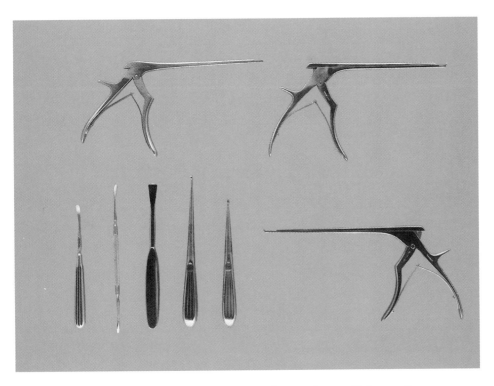

42-3 *Top, left to right,* 2 Kerrison rongeurs: 90 degree, 2 mm; 40 degree, 3 mm. *Bottom, left to right,* 1 Love Adson elevator (joker); 1 Freer elevator, double ended; 1 Langenbeck periosteal elevator; 2 Spratt curettes, No. 0: curved, 8 inch; straight, 6$\frac{1}{2}$ inch; 1 Kerrison rongeur, 40 degree, 2 mm.

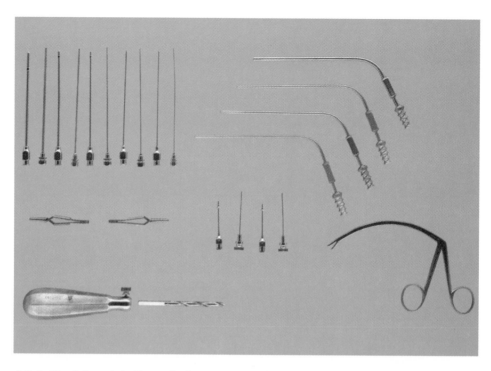

42-4 *Top left to right,* 5 ventricular needles with stylets, 3½ inch, 12, 14, 16, 18, and 20 gauge; 4 Frazier suction tubes, No. 3, 4, 6, and 8. *Middle, left to right,* 2 bulldog clips, straight, small; 2 Titus needles with stylets. *Bottom, left to right,* 1 hand drill handle; 1 drill bit; 1 Caroll tendon puller.

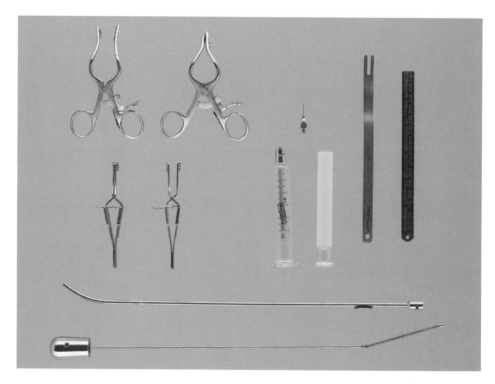

42-5 *Top left,* 2 Weitlaner retractors, angled, baby. *Middle, left to right,* 2 Heintz self-retaining retractors; 1 glass syringe with Luer-Lok, 10 ml; 1 Huber needle, 26 gauge; 1 Delta shunt tool; 1 metal ruler, 15 cm. *Bottom,* 1 salmon passer 14 inch, 2 parts.

43

Back Adds Instruments

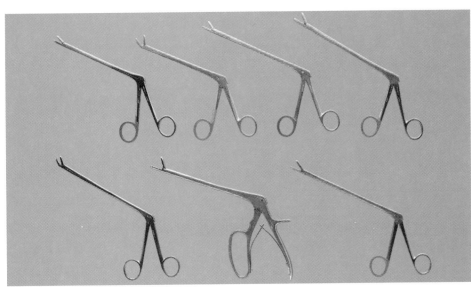

43-1 *Top left to right,* 4 Cushing intervertebral disc rongeur, 2 mm: straight, 6 inch; upbiting 6 inch; straight, 6 inch; straight, 7 inch. *Bottom, left to right,* 1 Cushing intervertebral disc rongeur, 3 mm, 7 inch, upbiting; 1 Ferris-Smith pituitary rongeur, 6 mm, 7 inch; 1 Cushing intervertebral disc rongeur, 4 mm, 7 inch.

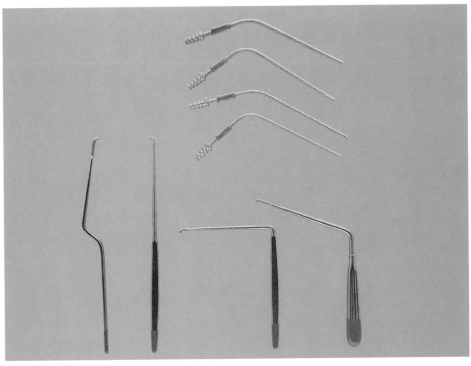

43-2 *Top to middle,* 4 Frazier suction tubes, 12, 10, 8, and 6 Fr. *Bottom, left to right,* 1 Derrico nerve root retractor; 1 Love nerve retractor, straight; 1 Love nerve retractor, right angle; 1 Scoville nerve root retractor.

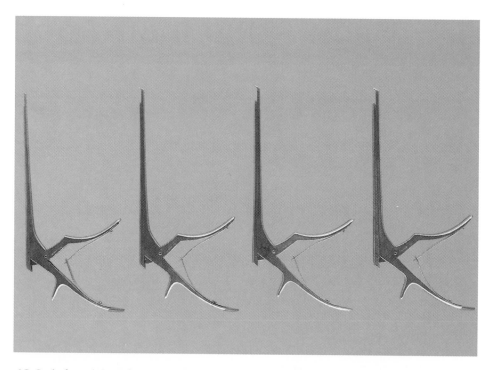

43-3 *Left to right,* 4 Spurling Kerrison rongeurs, 40 degree: 2, 3, 4, and 5 mm.

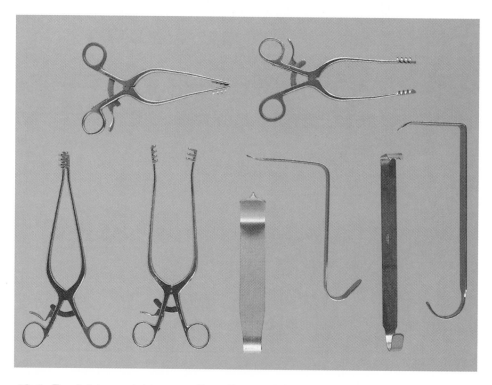

43-4 *Top,* 2 Adson retractors, medium. *Bottom, left to right,* 2 Weitlaner retractors, straight, long; 2 Taylor spinal retractors: short, front view; long, side view; 2 Hibbs laminectomy retractors: narrow, front view; wide, side view.

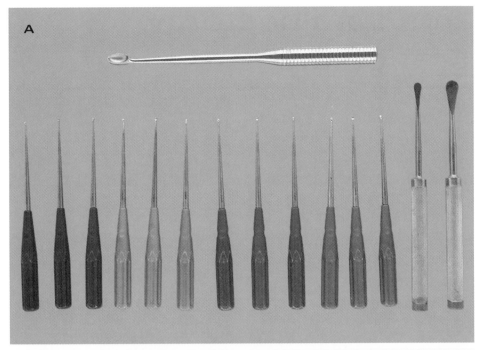

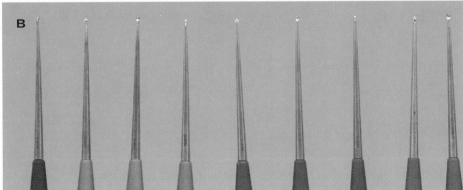

43-5 A, *Top,* 1 Mellon curette, long, large. *Bottom, left to right,* 3 curettes, size 4-0: reverse angled, angled, and straight; 3 curettes size, 2-0: reverse angled, angled, and straight; 3 curettes, size 3-0: reverse angled, angled, and straight; 3 curettes, size 0: reverse angled, angled, and straight; 2 Cobb spinal elevators, narrow, wide. **B,** *Left to right,* Curette tips: 1 4-0, straight; 3 2-0, reverse angled, angled, and straight; 3 3-0, reverse angled, angled, and straight; 2 0, reverse angled, and straight.

44

Williams Laminectomy Microretractors

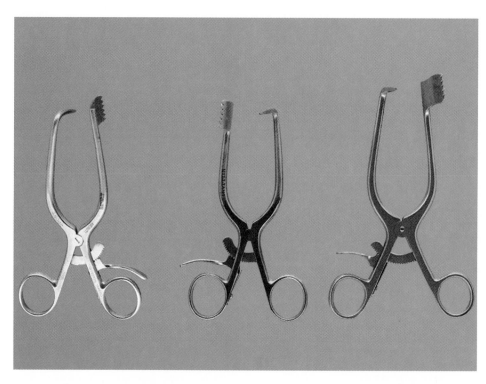

44-1 *Left to right,* Williams laminectomy microretractors: short blade, right handed, back side; long blade, right handed, front side; long blade, left handed, front side.

45

Anterior Cervical Fusion Set

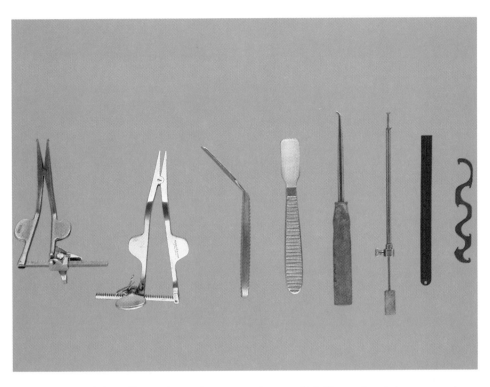

45-1 *Left to right,* 1 Cloward vertebrae spreader, small; 1 Cloward vertebrae spreader, medium; 2 Cloward blade retractors, modified, side view, front view; 1 osteophyte periosteal elevator; 1 depth gauge with set screw; 1 metal ruler; 1 Spanner wrench.

45-2 *Top, left to right,* 6 sets of blunt retractor blades, small to large. *Middle, left to right,* 1 Cloward retractor handle, small; 1 Cloward retractor handle, large. *Bottom, left to right,* 6 sets of 4 prong retractor blades, small to large.

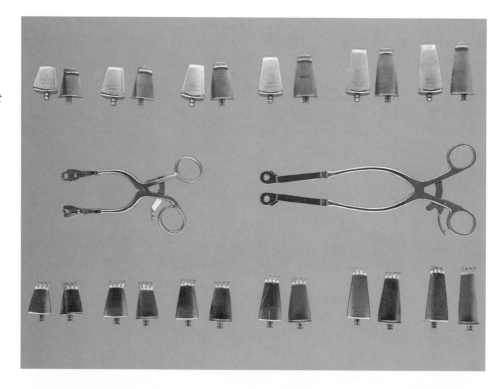

45-3 *Top, left to right,* 1 Hudson brace; 1 Dowel ejector. Bottom, left to right, 1 Dowel cutter shaft with removable threaded nut; 1 Cloward bone-graft double-ended impactor, $^{11}/_{14}$ mm; 1 Cloward drill shaft. *Middle, top to bottom,* 4 drill tips: 10, 12, 14, and 16 mm; 6 Dowel cutters with center pins, 12 to 18 mm; 4 Dowel cutters: 12, 14, 16, and 18 mm. *Bottom, right,* 1 Dowel handle, cone tip with spring.

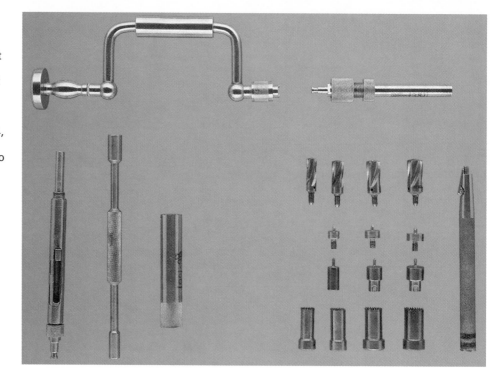

46

Caspar Set

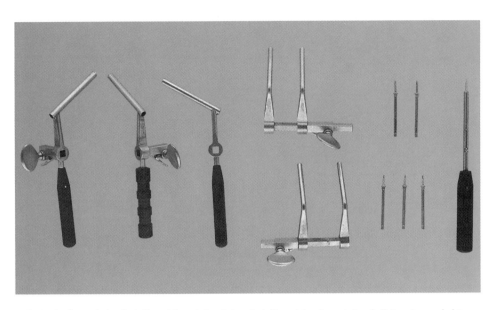

46-1 *Left to right,* 2 drill guides, left, right; 1 drill guide; 2 vertebral distractors, right, left; 5 distraction pins, 16 and 14 mm; 1 screwdriver.

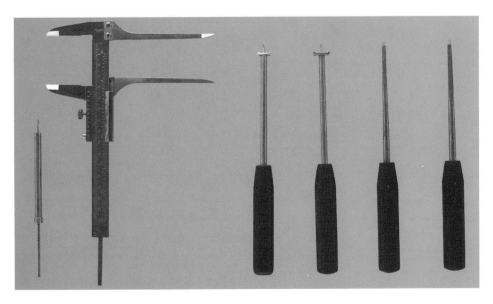

46-2 *Left to right,* 1 twist drill; 1 caliper; 1 vertebral body dissector; 1 vertebral body dissector, angled; 2 graft holders, small, standard.

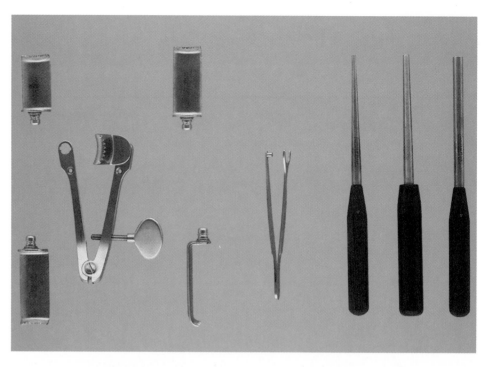

46-3 *Left to right,* Speculum pattern with 4 blades, 3 front view, 1 side view; blade ejector; 3 bone tamps, 3, 5, and 8 mm.

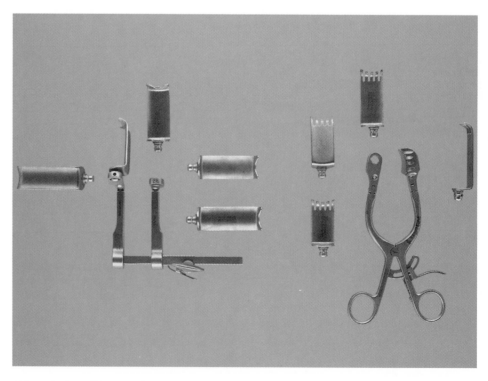

46-4 *Left to right,* vertebral distractor with 5 pins of various sizes; Caspar self-retaining retractor with 5 dull blades, 1 attached.

ASIF Anterior Cervical Locking Plating Instruments

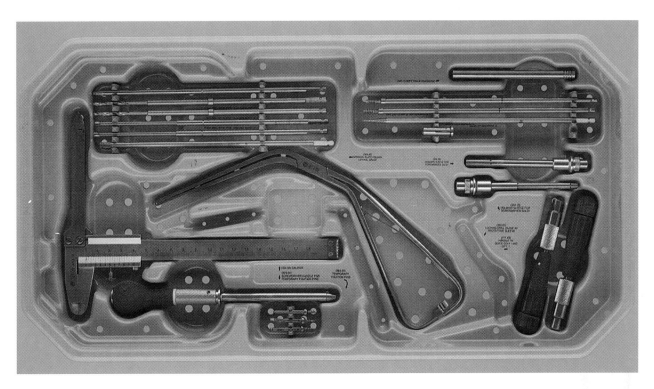

47-1 ASIF anterior cervical locking plating instruments in tray with names marked.

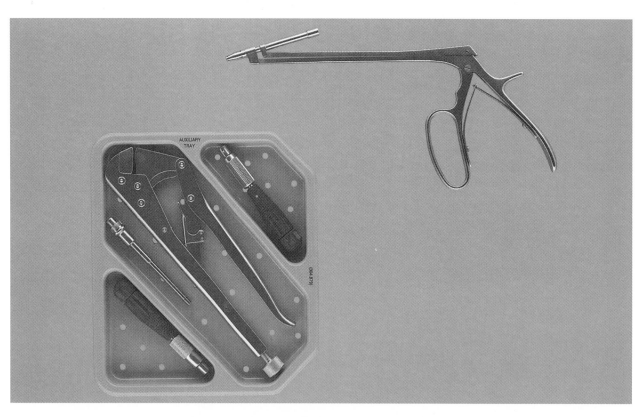

47-2 Drill guide with axillary bin, names marked.

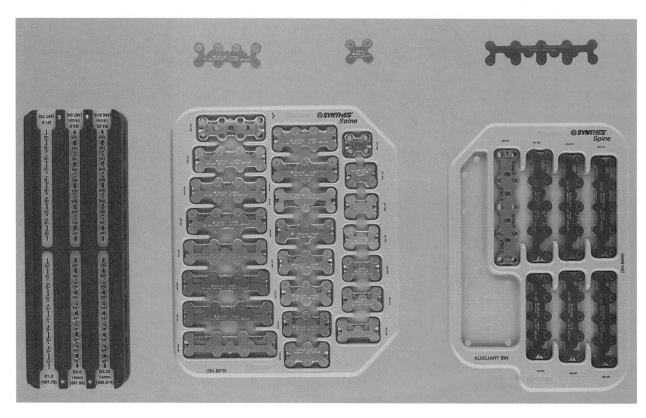

47-3 3 marked trays: 1 of screws and 2 of various sizers.

48

Midas Rex Drill

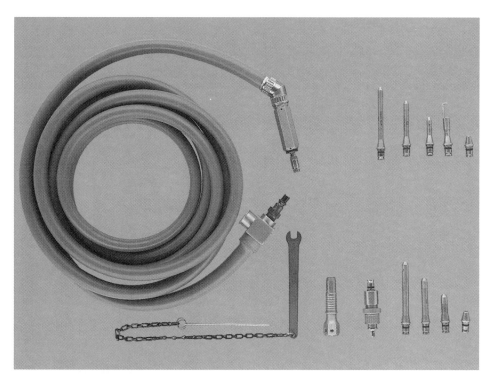

48-1 Midas Rex drill with power hose, wrench, chuck, and attachments.

49

Mednext Drill Assembly

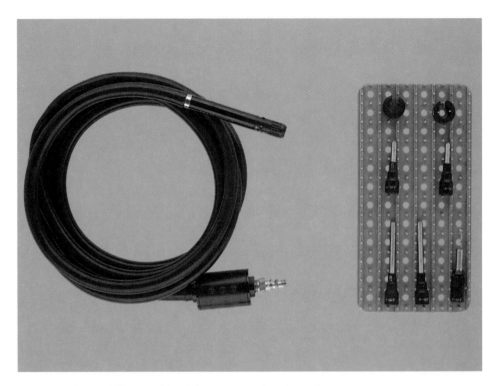

49-1 Mednext drill assembly with power cord and attachments.

50

ICP Monitoring Tray

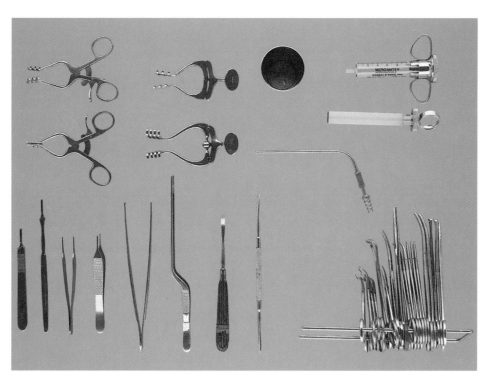

50-1 *Top, left to right,* 2 Weitlaner retractors, baby, front view, back view; 1 mastoid articulated retractor, 3 pronged; 1 Jansen retractor, 4 pronged; 1 metal medicine cup, 2 oz; 1 Frazier suction tube, 12 Fr; 1 Luer-Lok glass syringe with plunger and finger holds. *Bottom, left to right,* 2 Bard Parker knife handles, No. 3, No. 7; 2 Adson tissue forceps with teeth (1 × 2), front view, side view; 1 Cushing tissue forceps without teeth; 1 thumb dressing forceps, bayonet shaft; 1 Love-Adson (Cushing) periosteal elevator, curved tip; 1 Freer elevator; 5 Backhaus towel forceps, 4 small, 1 regular; 1 iris scissors, curved; 1 Metzenbaum scissors, 5 1/2 inch; 1 Mayo dissecting scissors, straight; 3 Halstead mosquito hemostatic forceps, curved; 3 Halstead mosquito hemostatic forceps, straight; 2 Mayo Pean hemostatic forceps, curved, 6 inch; 2 Allis tissue forceps; 1 Masson Mayo Hegar needle holder, 6 inch.

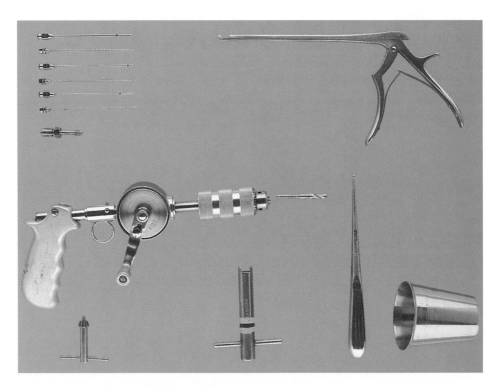

50-2 *Top, left to right,* 3 cone ventricular needles with stylets; 1 Richmond subarachnoid screw; 1 Spurling Kerrison rongeur, 40-degree angle, 3 mm. *Bottom, left to right,* 1 hand drill with bit; 1 chuck key; 1 Richmond subarachnoid wrench (T handle); 1 Spratt (Brun) curette, 3-0, small angle; 1 metal medicine cup, 8 oz.

Neuro Plating Instruments

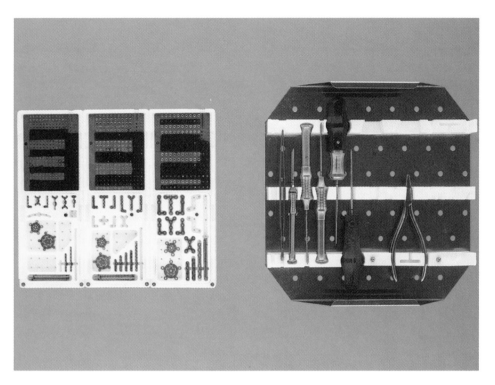

51-1 Neuro plating set: screws, plates, bur hole covers, drill bits, and instrumentation.

Yasargil Aneurysm Clips with Appliers

52-1 Yasargil aneurysm clips in marked tray.

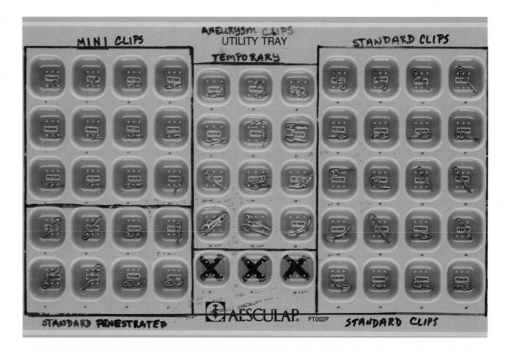

52-2 *Left, top to middle,* 2 Caspar appliers, angled: standard, mini-. *Bottom,* 2 bayonet clip appliers, standard, mini-. *Right, top to middle,* 2 Titan-Vario clip appliers, standard, mini-. *Middle,* 2 aneursym clips: silver, permanent; gold, temporary.

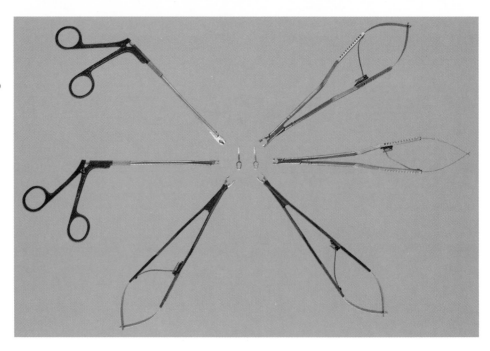

CUSA Handpieces

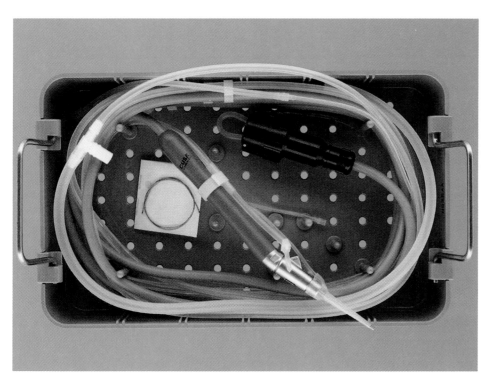

53-1 CUSA handpiece with attachments in tray.

54

Synthes Cranial Modular Fixation System—Maxillofacial

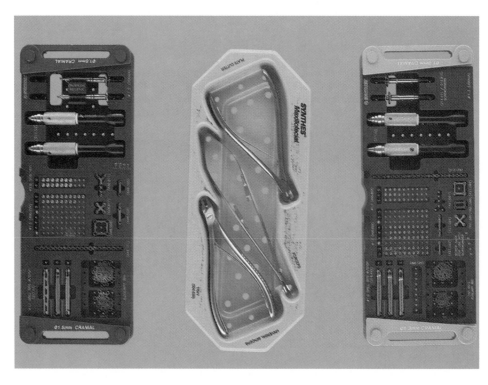

54-1 Synthes cranial modular fixation system (maxillofacial) in marked trays: 1.5 mm fixation system, instruments, 1.3 mm fixation system.

PERIPHERAL VASCULAR, CARDIOVASCULAR, AND THORACIC SURGERY

55

Peripheral Vascular Set

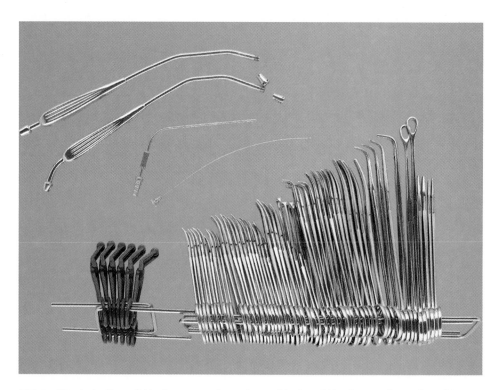

55-1 *Top to bottom,* 2 Yankauer suction tubes with tips; 1 Frazier suction tube with stylet. *Bottom, left to right,* 6 paper drape clips; 10 Halstead mosquito hemostatic forceps, curved; 6 Crile hemostatic forceps, curved, 5½ inch; 6 Providence hemostatic forceps (delicate tip), 5½ inch, curved; 4 Crile hemostatic forceps, curved, 6½ inch; 4 Allis tissue forceps; 4 Westphal hemostatic forceps; 6 tonsil hemostatic forceps; 2 Mayo Pean hemostatic forceps, long, curved; 2 Carmalt hemostatic forceps, long; 2 Adson hemostatic forceps, long; 2 Mixter hemostatic forceps, long, fine, and heavy tips; 2 Foerster sponge forceps; 2 Crile Wood needle holders, 7 inch; 2 Ayer needle holders, 7 inch, fine tips.

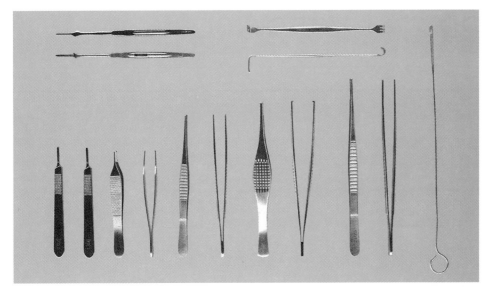

55-2 *Top, left to right,* 2 Bard Parker knife handles, No. 7; 2 Miller-Senn retractors. *Bottom, left to right,* 2 Bard Parker knife handles, No. 3; 2 Adson tissue forceps with teeth (1 × 2), side view, front view; 2 DeBakey Autraugrip tissue forceps, short, side view, front view; 2 Ferris-Smith tissue forceps, side view, front view; 2 DeBakey Autraugrip tissue forceps, medium, side view, front view; 1 eyed obturator (stylet) for Rumel tourniquet.

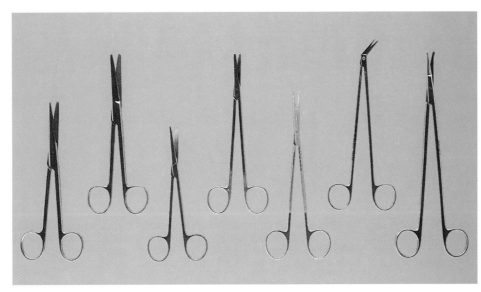

55-3 *Left to right,* 2 Mayo dissecting scissors, 1 straight, 1 curved; 2 Metzenbaum scissors, 5 inch, 7 inch; 1 Lincoln Metzenbaum scissors; 1 Potts-Smith cardiovascular scissors, 45-degree angle; 1 Strully scissors, probe tip.

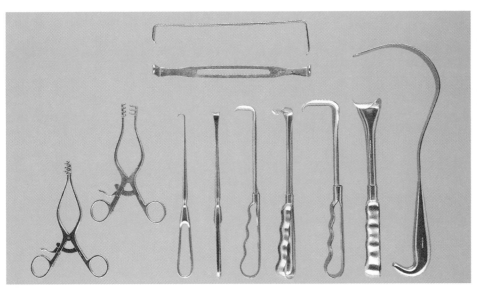

55-4 *Top,* 2 Army Navy retractors, side view, front view. *Bottom, left to right,* 2 Weitlaner retractors, sharp, medium; 2 vein retractors, side view, front view; 4 Richardson retractors, 2 small, 2 medium; 1 Deaver retractor, small.

56

Abdominal Vascular Set

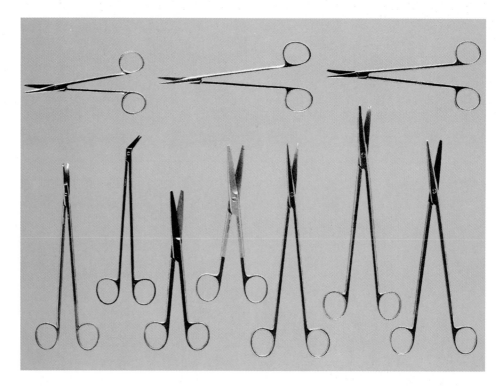

56-1 *Top, left to right,* 1 Metzenbaum scissors, 5 inch; 1 Lincoln Metzenbaum scissors; 1 Metzenbaum scissors, 7 inch. *Bottom, left to right,* 1 Strully scissors, probe tip; 1 Potts-Smith cardiovascular scissors, 45-degree angle; 2 Mayo dissecting scissors, straight; 1 Metzenbaum scissors, long, sharp; 2 Snowden-Pencer scissors, curved, straight.

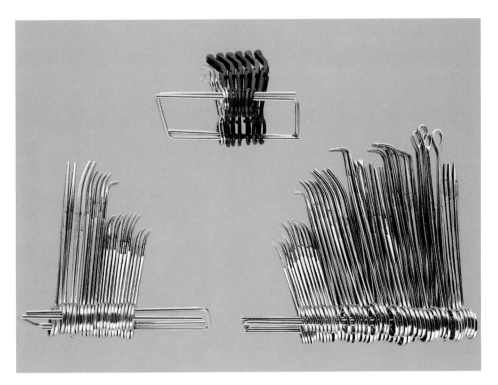

56-2 *Top, left to right,* 2 Backhaus towel forceps; 6 paper drape clips. *Bottom, left to right,* 2 Ochsner hemostatic forceps, straight, long; 2 Mayo Pean hemostatic forceps, long; 4 tonsil hemostatic forceps; 1 Westphal hemostatic forceps; 4 Providence hemostatic forceps (delicate tip), 5$\frac{1}{2}$ inch, curved; 4 Crile hemostatic forceps, curved, 5$\frac{1}{2}$ inch; 4 Halstead mosquito hemostatic forceps, curved. *Second stringer,* 4 Halstead mosquito hemostatic forceps, curved; 6 Crile hemostatic forceps, curved, 5$\frac{1}{2}$ inch; 1 Westphal hemostatic forceps; 4 tonsil hemostatic forceps; 4 Carmalt hemostatic forceps, long; 2 Adson hemostatic forceps, long; 2 Allis tissue forceps, long; 4 Ochsner hemostatic forceps, long, straight; 3 Mixter hemostatic forceps, long, heavy tip; 2 Mixter hemostatic forceps, long, fine tipped; 4 Foerster sponge forceps; 2 Ayer needle holders, 8 inch; 2 Crile Wood needle holders, 8 inch.

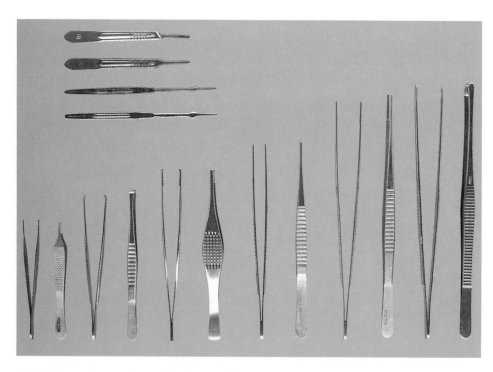

56-3 *Top to bottom,* 4 Bard Parker needle holders, 2 No. 4, 2 No. 7. *Bottom,* 2 Adson tissue forceps with teeth (1 × 2), front view, side view; 2 Hayes Martin tissue forceps with multiteeth, short, front view, side view; 2 Ferris-Smith tissue forceps, front view, side view; 4 DeBakey Autraugrip tissue forceps, 2 medium, 2 long, front view, side view; 2 Russian tissue forceps, long, front view, side view.

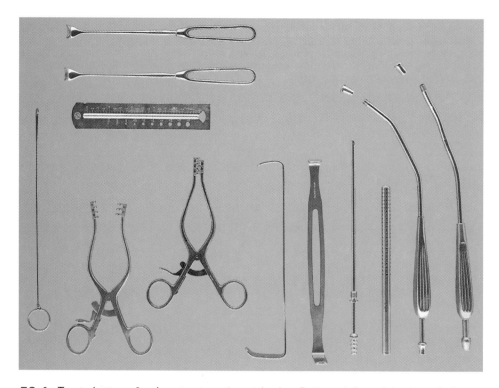

56-4 *Top to bottom,* 2 vein retractors; 1 metal ruler. *Bottom, left to right,* 1 eyed obturator (stylet) for Rumel tourniquet; 2 Weitlaner retractors, sharp, medium; 2 Army Navy retractors, side view, front view; 1 Poole abdominal suction tube with shield; 2 Yankauer suction tubes with tips.

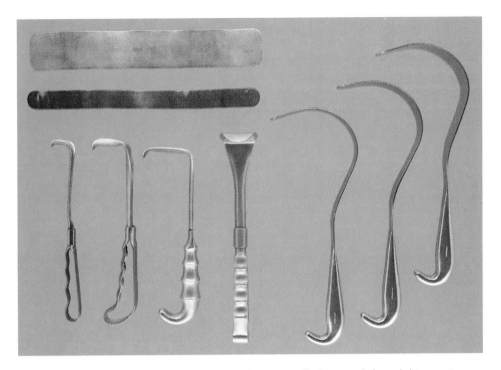

56-5 *Top,* 2 Ochsner malleable retractors, large, small. *Bottom, left to right,* 4 Richardson retractors, 1 small, 1 medium, 2 large, side view, front view; 3 Deaver retractors, small, medium, large.

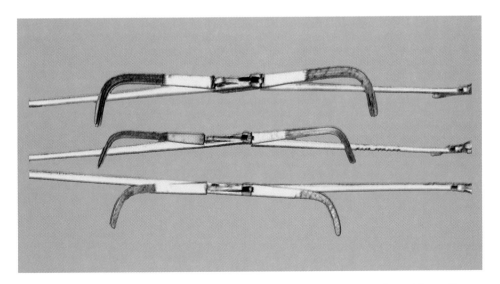

56-6 *Top to bottom,* Tips: 2 Mixter hemostatic forceps, long, heavy tip and long, fine tip; Adson hemostatic forceps.

57

Basic Open Heart Set

ADD OPEN HEART EXTRAS

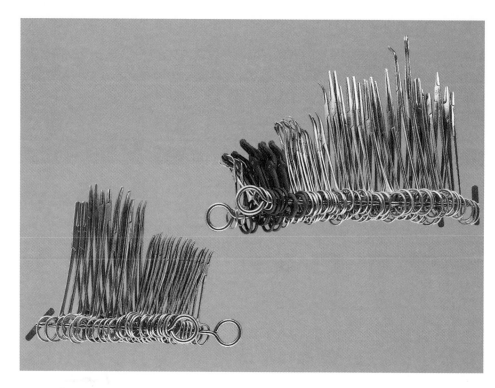

57-1 *Bottom, left,* 5 Halstead mosquito hemostatic forceps, curved; 10 Crile hemostatic forceps, 5$\frac{1}{2}$ inch; 4 tonsil hemostatic forceps, blunt tipped; 2 Mayo Pean hemostatic forceps, long; 2 Ayer needle holders, 8 inch; 1 DeBakey needle holder, 8 inch; 1 Crile Wood needle holder, 8 inch; 2 Vorse-Webster tubing occluding clamps. *Top, right,* 2 Backhaus towel forceps, small; 8 paper drape clips; 3 Peers towel forceps, blunt tipped; 3 Backhaus towel forceps; 4 Providence hemostatic forceps, delicate tipped; 3 Crile hemostatic forceps, 5$\frac{1}{2}$ inch; 1 Adson hemostatic forceps, curved; 2 Ochsner hemostatic forceps, straight, short jawed; 10 Ochsner hemostatic forceps, straight, medium jawed; 1 Mixter hemostatic forceps, long; 1 Foerster sponge forceps; 2 Vorse-Webster tubing occluding clamps; 1 Berry sternal needle holder (short jawed); 3 Crile Wood needle holders, 1 8 inch, 2 7 inch.

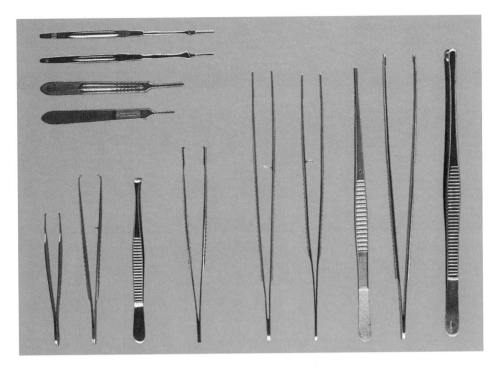

57-2 *Top, left,* 4 Bard Parker knife handles, 2 No. 7, 1 No. 4, 1 No. 3. *Bottom, left to right,* 1 Adson tissue forceps with teeth (1 × 2); 2 Hayes Martin tissue forceps with multiteeth, front view, side view; 1 Ferris-Smith tissue forceps; 3 DeBakey Autraugrip tissue forceps with post, long, 2 front views, 1 side view; 2 Russian tissue forceps, long, front view, side view.

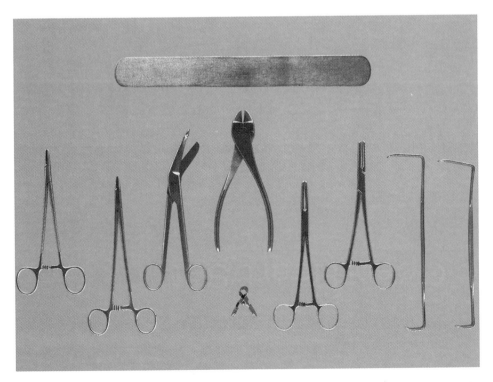

57-3 *Top,* 1 Ochsner malleable retractor, medium. *Bottom, left to right,* 2 Berry sternal needle holders, 7 inch, 8 inch; 1 bandage scissors, heavy; 1 wire cutter, heavy; 1 bed cord-holding clip; 2 Vorse-Webster tubing occluding clamps; 2 Army Navy retractors.

57-4 *Left to right,*
1 DeBakey multipurpose
vascular clamp, obtuse
angle, 60 degrees, jaw
length 4 cm, overall length
9 inches; 1 Glover patent
ductus clamp, straight;
1 Beck aorta clamp; 2 eyed
obturators (stylets) for
Rumel tourniquet;
2 Yankauer suction tubes
with tips.

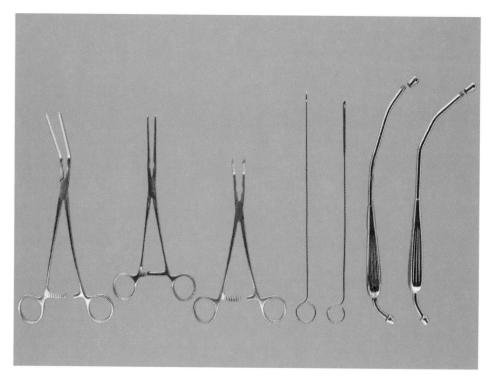

57-5 *Top,* 3 Hegar dilators, 7 and 8, 5 and 6, 3 and
4. *Bottom, left to right,*
4 Mayo dissecting scissors,
1 curved, 3 straight;
3 Metzenbaum scissors,
2 7 inch, 1 8 inch; 1 Strully
scissors with probe tip.

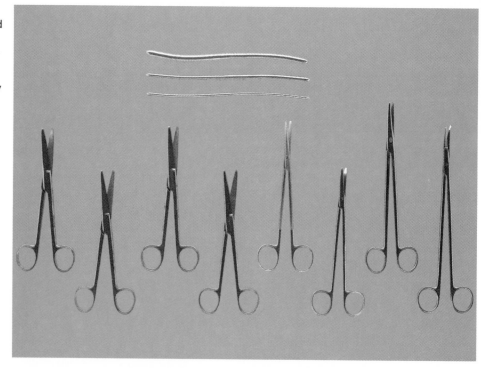

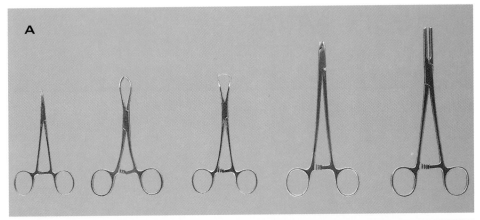

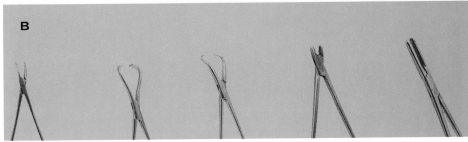

57-6 **A**, *Left to right,* Providence hemostatic forceps, curved, delicate tipped; Peers towel forceps, blunt; Backhaus towel forceps; Berry sternal needle holder; Vorse-Webster tubing-occluding clamp. **B**, *Left to right,* Tips: Providence hemostatic forceps, curved, delicate tipped; Peers towel forceps, blunt; Backhaus towel forceps; Berry sternal needle holder; Vorse-Webster tubing-occluding clamp.

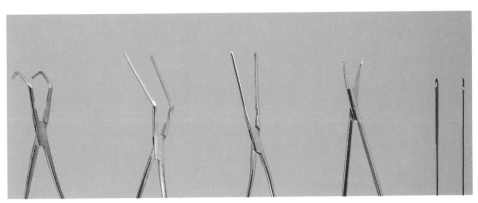

57-7 *Left to right,* Tips: Beck aorta clamp; DeBakey multipurpose vascular clamp, obtuse angle, 60 degrees, jaw length 4 cm; Glover patent ductus clamp, straight; Strulley scissors; eyed obturator (stylet) for Rumel tourniquet.

58

Open Heart Micro Instruments

ADD BASIC OPEN HEART SET AND OPEN HEART EXTRAS

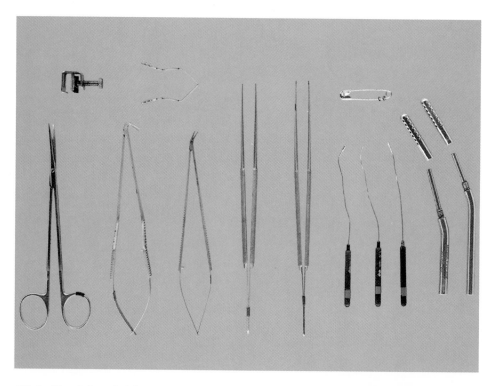

58-1 *Top, left and right,* 1 tubing clamp; 1 Parsonnet epicardial (self-retaining spring) retractor; 1 safety pin with rings. *Bottom, left to right,* 1 Snowden-Pencer scissors, straight; 1 Snowden-Pencer micro–needle holder, curved; 1 Snowden-Pencer microscissors, curved; 2 Snowden-Pencer dressing forceps, 8 inch; 3 Garrett dilators, graduated sizes; 2 metal coronary suction tubes with tips.

Open Heart Extras

ADD BASIC OPEN HEART SET

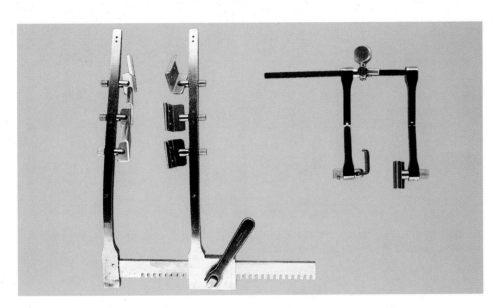

59-1 *Left to right,* 1 Ankeney sternal retractor; 1 Himmelstein sternal retractor.

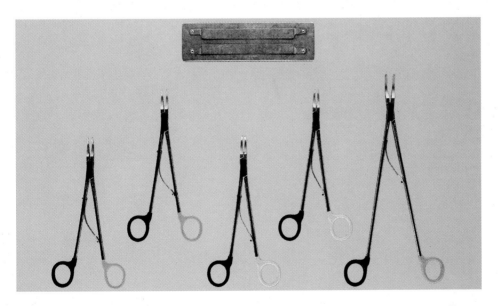

59-2 *Top,* 1 hemoclip cartridge base. *Bottom, left to right,* 5 Weck EZ load hemoclip appliers: 2 medium, 7.75 inch; 2 small, 7.75 inch; 1 large, 10.75 inch.

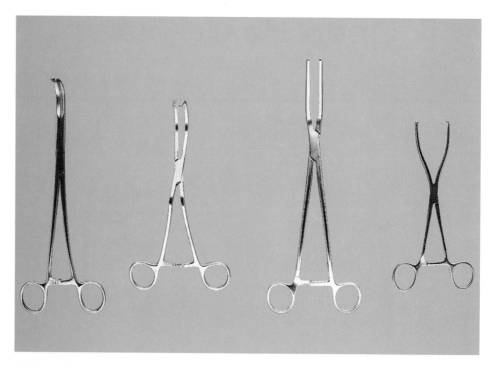

59-3 *Left to right,* 1 Semb dissecting forceps; 1 Lampert-Kay clamp; 1 Fogarty clamp-applying forceps, angled; 1 bulldog applier.

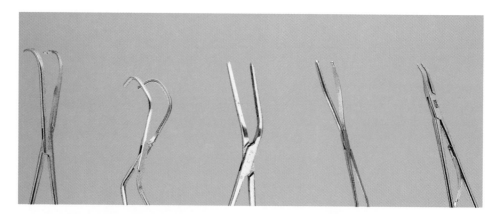

59-4 *Left to right,* Tips: 1 Semb dissecting forceps; 1 Lampert-Kay clamp; 1 Fogarty clamp-applying forceps, angled; 1 bulldog applier; 1 Weck EZ load hemoclip appliers, medium.

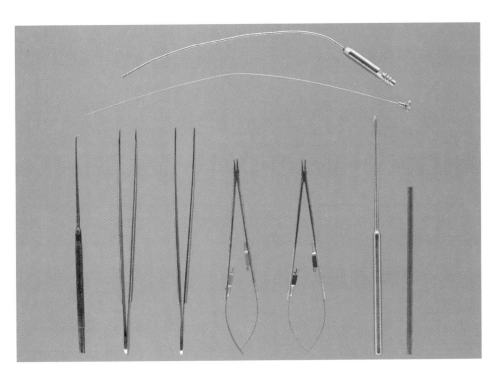

59-5 *Top,* 1 Frazier suction tube with stylet, long. *Bottom, left to right,* 1 Adson dissector hook; 2 Ruel dressing forceps; 2 Castroviejo needle holders with locks, 7 inch; 1 Penfield dissector, single-ended, No. 4; 1 Beaver knife handle, knurled, 6 inch, without insert.

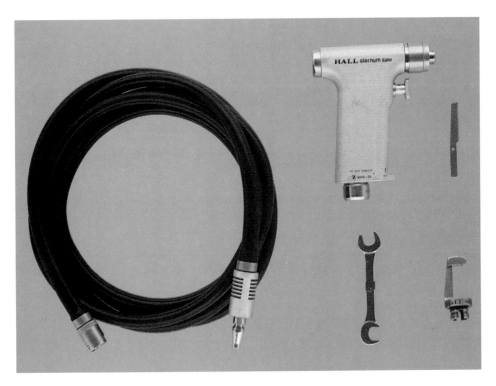

59-6 Hall sternal saw, power hose, wrench, blade, saw guide.

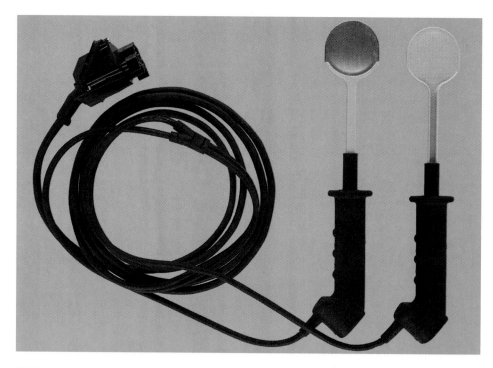

59-7 Internal defibulator paddles with power cord.

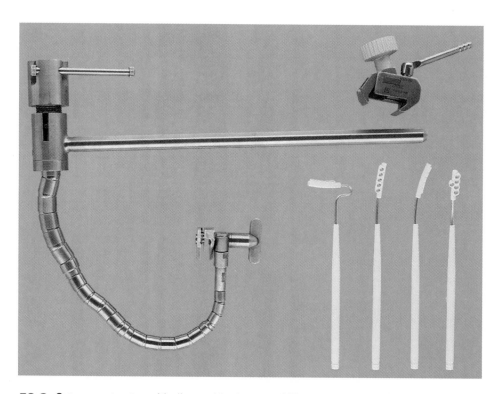

59-8 Octopus retractor with disposable tissue stabilizers.

Cardiovascular Instruments

ADD BASIC OPEN HEART SET

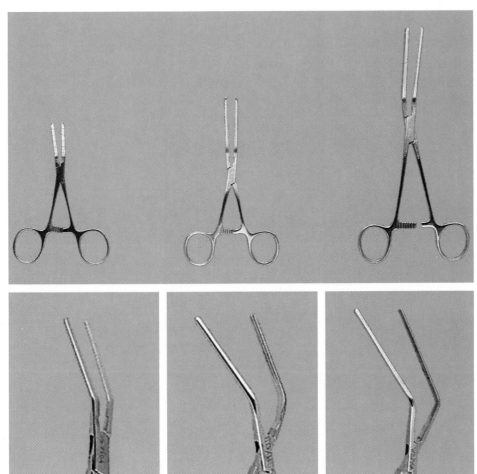

60-1 *Left to right,* 2 pediatric bulldog clamps: front view, tip; 2 DeBakey bulldog clamps: front view, tip; 2 DeBakey peripheral vascular clamps, front view, tip.

60-2 *Left to right,*
2 Fogarty clamp-applying forceps, angled: front view, tip; 2 Fogarty clamp-applying forceps, straight: front view, tip; 2 Cooley renal clamps: front view, tip.

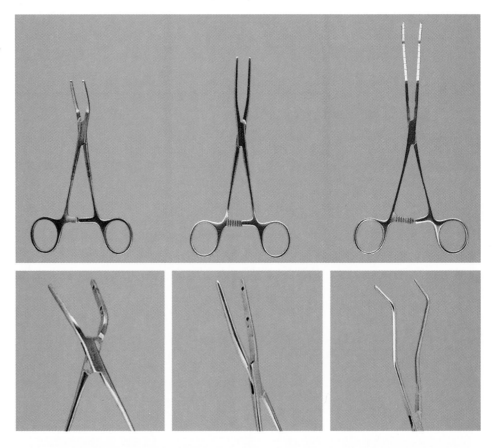

60-3 *Left to right,*
2 Snowden-Pencer tissue forceps, short: front view, tip; 2 Lee bronchus clamps: front view, tip; 2 coarctation clamps, angled handles: front view, tip.

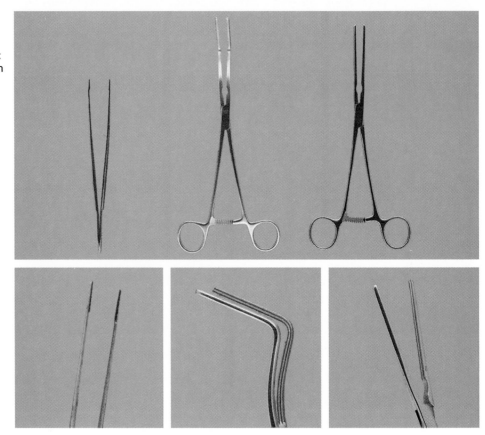

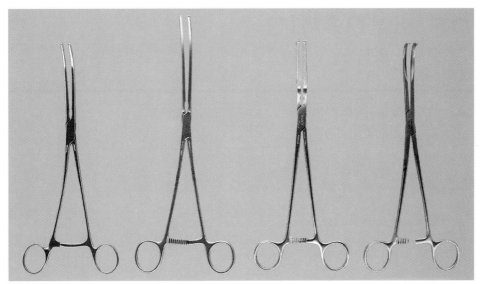

60-4 *Left to right,* 2 DeBakey aortic occlusion clamp, curved: medium, long; 1 DeBakey multipurpose vascular clamp, obtuse angle, 60 degrees; 1 Semb dissecting forceps.

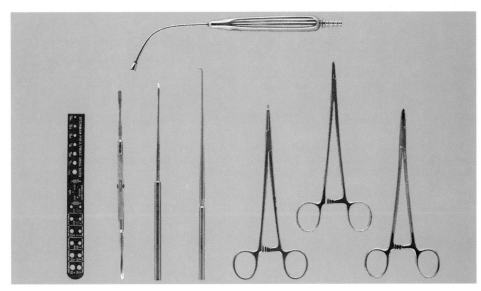

60-5 *Top,* 1 Andrews Pynchon suction tube. *Bottom, left to right,* 1 metal ruler, 6 inch; 1 Freer double-ended elevator; 1 Penfield dissector, single-ended, No. 4; 1 Hoen nerve hook; 1 Adson hemostatic forceps, angled, fine tipped; 2 Ryder needle holders, 7 inch, fine tipped.

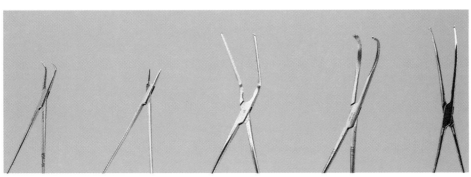

60-6 *Left to right,* Tips: 1 Adson hemostatic forceps, angled, fine tipped; 1 Ryder needle holders, fine tipped; 1 DeBakey multipurpose vascular clamp, obtuse angle, 60 degrees, jaw length 4 cm; 1 Semb dissecting forceps; 1 DeBakey aortic occlusion clamp, curved.

61

Rib Instruments

ADD ABDOMINAL VASCULAR SET AND CARDIOVASCULAR INSTRUMENTS

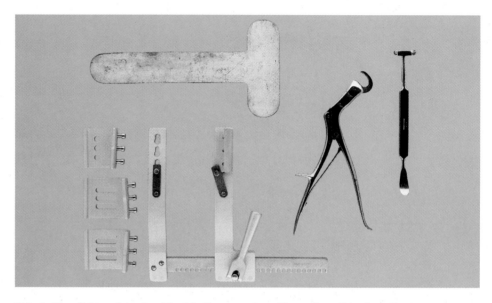

61-1 *Top, left to right,* 1 malleable T retractor; 1 Giertz (first rib) (rib guillotine) rongeur; 1 Matson rib stripper and elevator. *Bottom left,* 1 Burford rib spreader with shallow blade attached: 1 shallow blade, 2 deep blades.

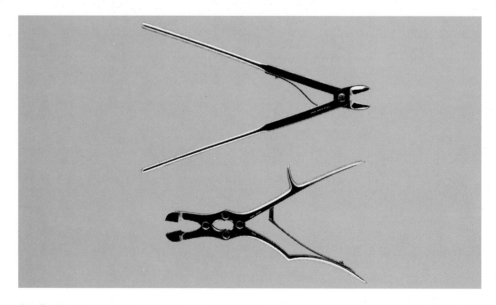

61-2 *Top to bottom,* 1 Bethune (rib) rongeur; 1 Sauerbruch (rib) rongeur, double action.

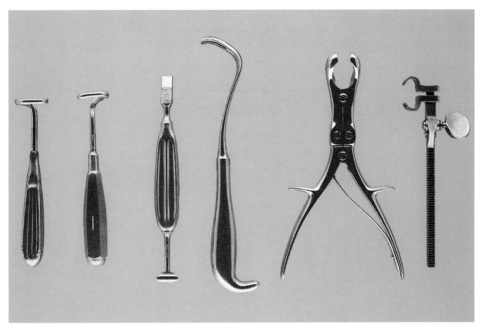

61-3 *Left to right,* 2 Doyen rib elevators and raspatories, left, right; 1 Alexander rib raspatory (periosteotome), double ended; 1 Semb lung retractor; 1 Semb gouging rongeur, double action; 1 Bailey rib contractor

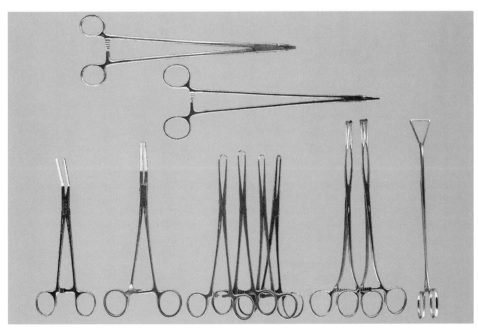

61-4 *Top,* 2 Crile Wood needle holders, 11 inch. *Bottom, left to right,* 1 Potts bronchus forceps, 25-degree angle; 1 DeBakey bronchus forceps, angular; 4 Allis tissue forceps, long; 3 Duval Crile tissue forceps, 2 front views, 1 side view.

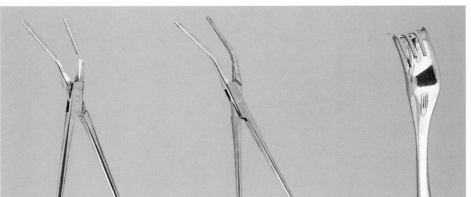

61-5 *Left to right,* Tips: 1 Potts bronchus forceps, 25-degree angle; 1 DeBakey bronchus forceps, angular; 1 Semb lung retractor.

62

Open Heart Valve Extras

ADD BASIC OPEN HEART SET AND OPEN HEART EXTRAS AS NEEDED

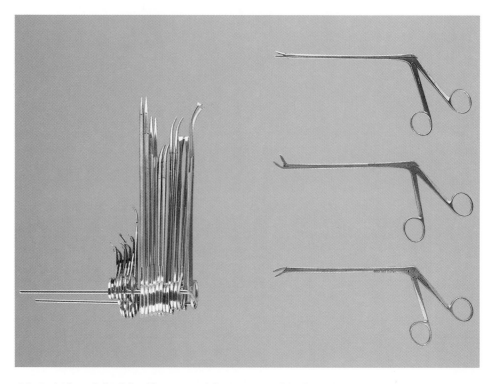

62-1 *Left to right,* 6 Backhaus towel forceps, small; 1 Providence hemostatic forceps; 2 Ayer needle holders, 11 inch; 2 Heaney needle holders; 2 tonsil hemostatic forceps; 2 tonsil hemostatic forceps, long; 2 Allis tissue forceps, long; 1 Allis tissue forceps, long, curved. *Top to bottom,* 1 pituitary rongeur, straight bite, 7 inch; 1 pituitary rongeur, upbite, 7 inch; 1 pituitary rongeur, downbite, 7 inch.

168

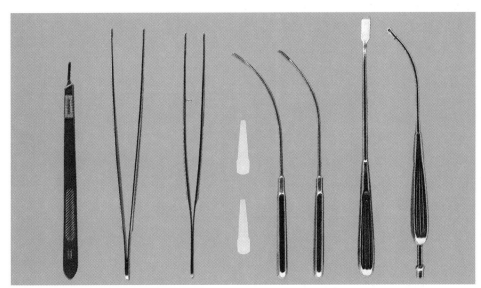

62-2 *Left to right,* 1 Bard Parker knife handle, No. 3, long; 1 Brown Adson tissue forceps with teeth (7 × 7); 1 Cushing tissue forceps with teeth (1 × 2); 2 teflon bardic plugs; 3 leaflet retractors: 2 side views, 1 front view; 1 Andrews Pynchon suction tube.

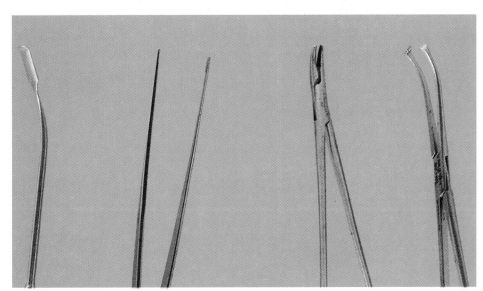

62-3 *Left to right,* Tips: 1 leaflet retractor; 1 Brown Adson tissue forceps with teeth (7 × 7); Heaney needle holder; 1 Allis tissue forceps, curved.

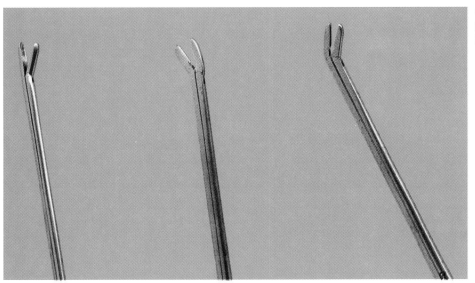

62-4 *Left to right,* 3 pituitary rongeurs tips: straight bite, downbite, upbite.

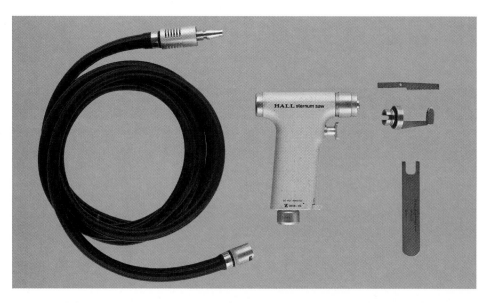

63-1 *Left to right,* Power cord; Hall sternum saw. *Top to bottom,* 1 saw blade; 1 saw guide; 1 wrench.

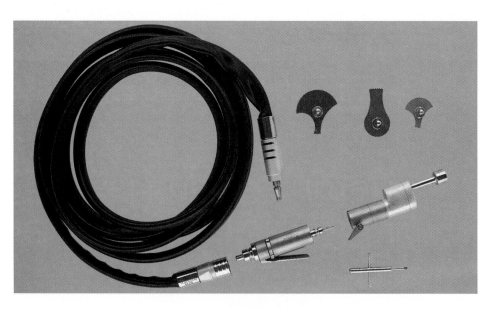

63-2 *Left to right,* Power cord. *Top to bottom,* 3 saw blades; Aesculap oscillating sternal saw, 2 parts; 1 wrench.

Return Open Heart Set

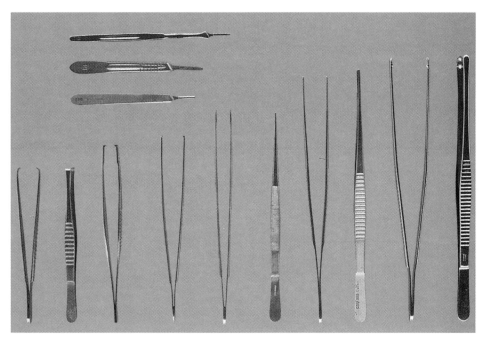

64-1 *Top left,* 3 Bard Parker knife handles: 1 No. 7, 1 No. 4, 1 No. 3. *Bottom, left to right,* 2 Hayes Martin tissue forceps with multi-teeth, front view, side view; 1 Ferris-Smith tissue forceps; 1 Cushing tissue forceps with teeth (1 × 2), 7 inch; 2 Ruel dressing forceps, front view, side view; 2 DeBakey Autraugrip tissue forceps, long, front view, side view; 2 Russian tissue forceps, long, front view, side view.

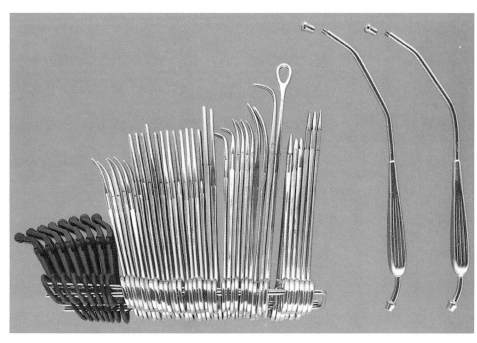

64-2 *Left to right,* 8 paper drape clips; 6 Crile hemostatic forceps, 6½ inch; 12 Ochsner hemostatic forceps, medium jaw; 2 Ochsner hemostatic forceps, long jaw; 2 Westphal hemostatic forceps, short; 4 tonsil hemostatic forceps; 2 Mayo Pean hemostatic forceps, long, curved; 1 Adson hemostatic forceps, long; 1 Foerster sponge forceps; 1 Crile Wood needle holder, 7 inch; 2 Berry sternal needle holders, 7 inch; 2 Crile Wood needle holders, 8 inch; 1 Ayer needle holder, 8 inch; 2 Yankauer suction tubes with tips.

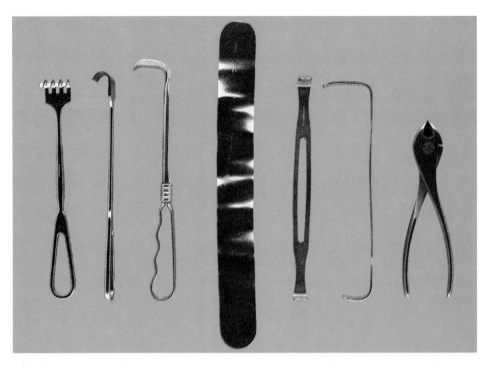

64-3 *Left to right,* 2 Volkmann retractors, 4 prong, dull, front view, side view; 1 Richardson retractor, small; 1 Ochsner malleable retractor, medium; 2 Army Navy retractors, front view, side view; 1 wire cutter, heavy.

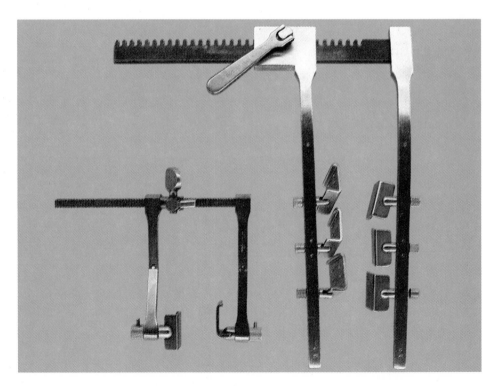

64-4 *Left to right,* 1 Himmelstein sternal retractor; 1 Ankeney sternal retractor.

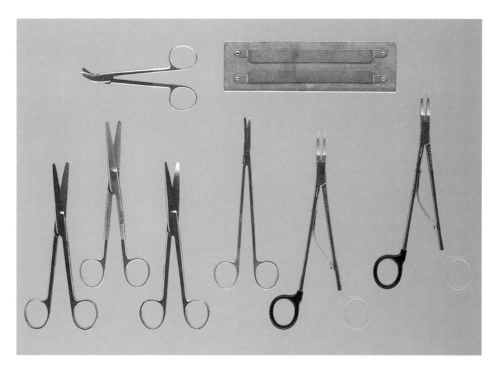

64-5 *Top, left to right,* 1 wire cutter, small; 1 hemoclip cartridge base. *Bottom, left to right,* 3 Mayo dissecting scissors: 2 straight, 1 curved; 1 Metzenbaum scissors, 7 inch; 2 Weck EZ load hemoclip appliers.

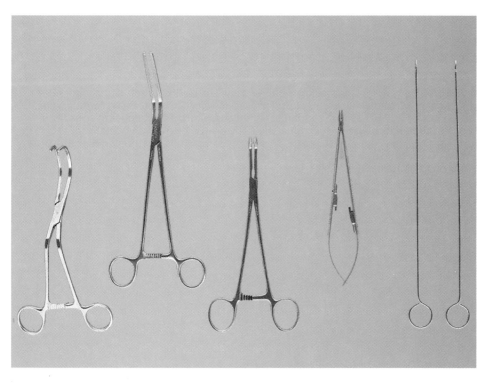

64-6 *Left to right,* 1 Lambert-Kay clamp; 1 DeBakey multipurpose vascular clamp, obtuse angle, 60 degrees; 1 Beck aorta clamp; 1 Castroviejo needle holder with lock 7 inch; 2 eyed obturators (stylets) for Rumel tourniquet.

65

Vein Retrieval Instruments

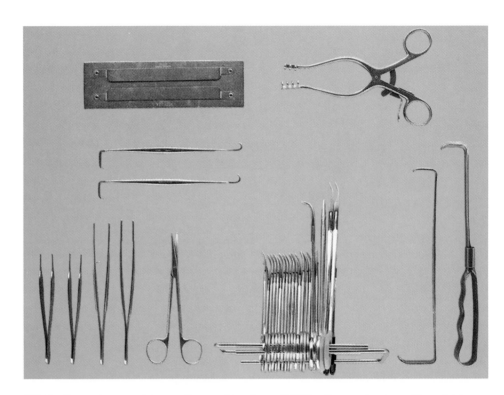

65-1 *Top to bottom,* 1 hemoclip cartridge base; 2 Miller-Senn retractors. *Top, right,* 1 Weitlaner retractor, sharp, small. *Bottom, left to right,* 2 Adson tissue forceps with teeth (1 × 2); 2 DeBakey Autraugrip tissue forceps, short; 1 Metzenbaum scissors, 5 inch; 10 Providence hemostatic forceps; 4 Halstead mosquito hemostatic forceps, curved; 1 Westphal hemostatic forceps, short; 1 Johnson needle holder, 5 inch; 1 Crile Wood needle holder, 7 inch; 2 Weck EZ load hemoclip appliers, medium; 1 Army Navy retractor; 1 Richardson retractor, small.

EYE, EAR, NOSE, AND THROAT SURGERY

66

Basic Eye Set

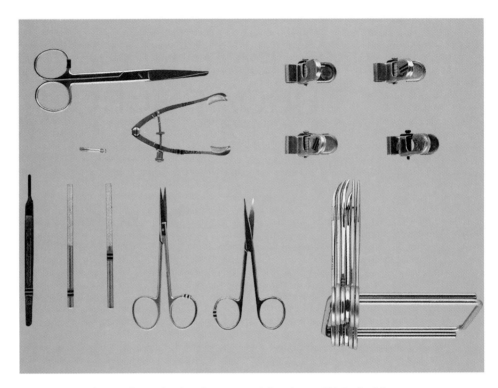

66-1 *Top, left to right,* 1 plastic scissors, straight, sharp, 5½ inch; 1 Lancaster speculum; 4 Edwards holding clips. *Bottom, left to right,* 1 Bard Parker knife handle, No. 9; 2 Beaver knife handles, knurled, one insert above; 1 Stevens tenotomy scissors, curved, blunt; 1 iris scissors, straight, 4½ inch; 6 Halstead mosquito hemostatic forceps, 4 curved, 2 straight.

67

Cataract Instruments

ADD BASIC EYE SET, INTRAOCULAR, AND MICROEYE INSTRUMENTS

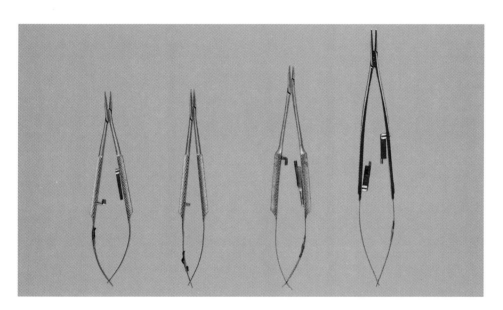

67-1 *Left to right,* 2 titanium micro–needle holders, curved: with lock, without lock; 1 Troutman Barraquer micro–needle holder, curved, with lock; 1 Castroviejo needle holder, straight, with lock.

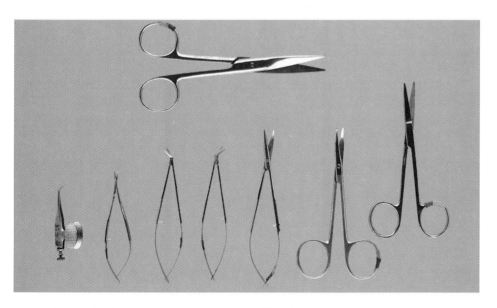

67-2 *Top,* 1 plastic scissors, straight, sharp, 5^1/$_2$ inch. *Bottom, left to right,* 1 Barraquer iris scissors, short; 1 Vannas capsulotomy scissors; 2 Castroviejo corneal section scissors, left, right; 1 Westcott tenotomy scissors; 1 Stevens tenotomy scissors, curved; 1 iris scissors, straight, 4^1/$_2$ inch.

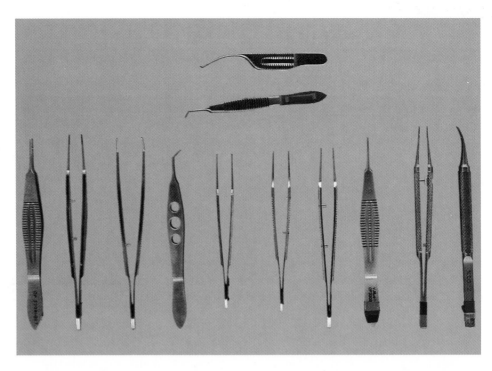

67-3 *Top to bottom,* 1 Colibrí corneal utility forceps, 0.4 mm, teeth (1 × 2), side view; 1 Kelman-McPherson tying forceps, narrow handles, side view. *Bottom, left to right,* 2 Castroviejo suturing forceps, wide handles, without tying platforms, 0.12 mm teeth (1 × 2), side view, front view; 1 Castroviejo suturing forceps, wide handles, without tying platforms, 0.5 mm teeth (1 × 2), front view; 1 Kelman-McPherson tying forceps, angled, side view, wide handles; 1 Bishop-Harmon tissue forceps; 1 McPherson tying forceps, straight; 2 Castroviejo suturing forceps, wide handles, with tying platforms, 0.5 mm teeth (1 × 2), front view, side view; 2 Troutman superior rectus forceps, front view, side view.

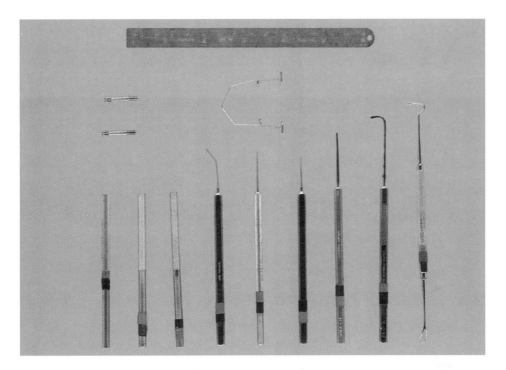

67-4 *Middle, top to bottom,* 1 metal ruler; 1 Barraquer wire speculum. *Left to right,* 3 Beaver knife handles, knurled with 2 inserts above; 1 Sinskey hook; 1 Jaffee lens spatula, straight; 1 Graether ocular button; 1 iris spatula; 1 Graefe muscle hook; 1 Kirby hook and loop.

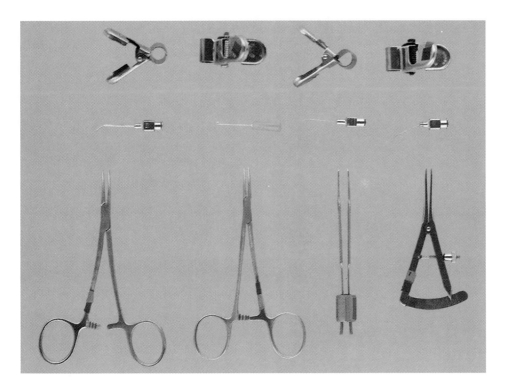

67-5 *Top to bottom,* 4 Edwards holding clips; 4 irrigating cannulas with various tips. *Bottom, left to right,* 2 Halstead mosquito hemostatic forceps, curved; 1 bipolar forceps; 1 Castroviejo caliper.

68

Eye Muscle Instruments

ADD BASIC EYE SET

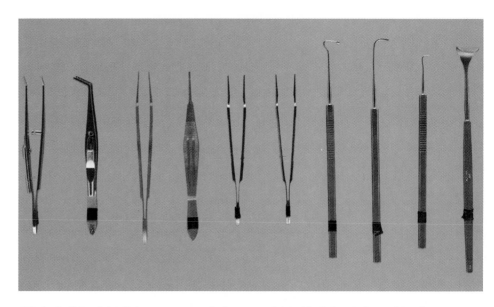

68-1 *Left to right,* 2 Jameson muscle forceps, right-sided, front view, side view; 2 Castroviejo suturing forceps, wide handles, without tying platforms, 0.5 mm teeth (1 × 2), front view, side view; 2 McCullough utility forceps; 1 Jameson strabismus hook; 1 Graefe muscle hook; 1 Stevens tenotomy hook; 1 Desmarres lid retractor.

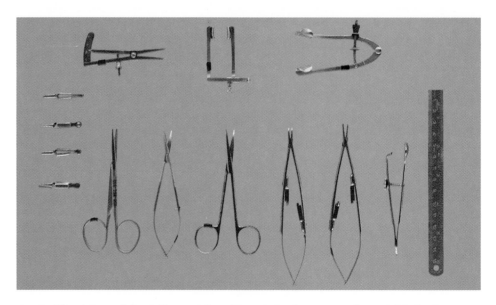

68-2 *Top, left to right,* 1 Castroviejo caliper; 1 Cook eye speculum, child sized; 1 Lancaster speculum. *Bottom, left to right,* 4 serrefines; 1 strabismus scissors, straight; 1 Westcott tenotomy scissors; 1 Stevens tenotomy scissors, curved; 2 Castroviejo needle holders with locks, curved, straight; 1 Erhardt chalazion clamp; 1 metal ruler, small.

69

Retinal Instruments

ADD BASIC EYE SET

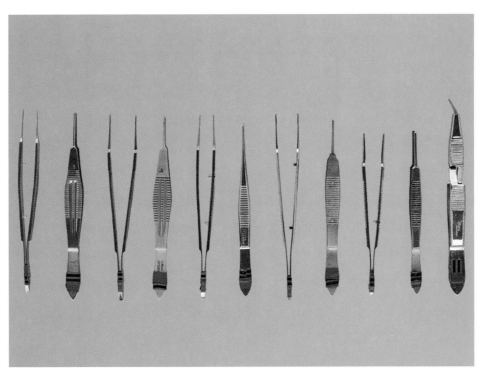

69-1 *Left to right,* 4 Castroviejo suturing forceps, wide handles, with tying platforms: 1 at 0.3 mm, 2 at 0.5 mm, 1 at 0.12 mm, front view, side view; 1 Troutman tying forceps; 1 Elschnig fixation forceps; 1 Harms tying forceps; 1 serrated forceps, straight; 2 McCullough utility forceps; 1 Watzke sleeve spreader forceps.

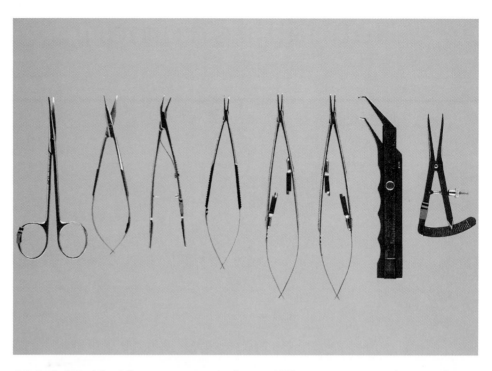

69-2 *Left to right,* 1 Stevens tenotomy scissors; 1 Westcott tenotomy scissors; 1 Green needle holder and forceps; 3 Castroviejo needle holders, straight; 1 without lock, 2 with locks; 1 Thorpe caliper; 1 Castroviejo caliper.

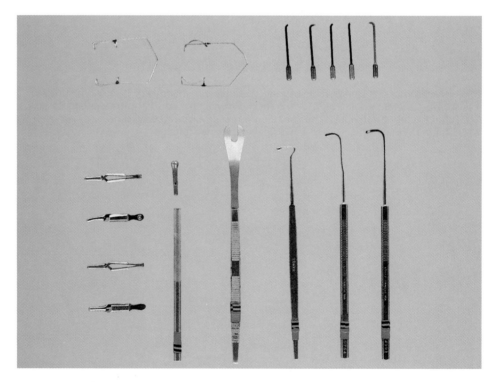

69-3 *Top, left to right,* 2 Barraquer wire speculums; 5 diathermy tips, Mira, assorted. *Bottom, left to right,* 4 serrefines; 1 Beaver knife handle, knurled, with insert above; 1 Schepens orbital retractor; 1 Jameson strabismus hook; 1 Graefe muscle hook; 1 Gass hook.

Intraocular Instruments

ADD BASIC CATARACT INSTRUMENTS AND BASIC EYE SET

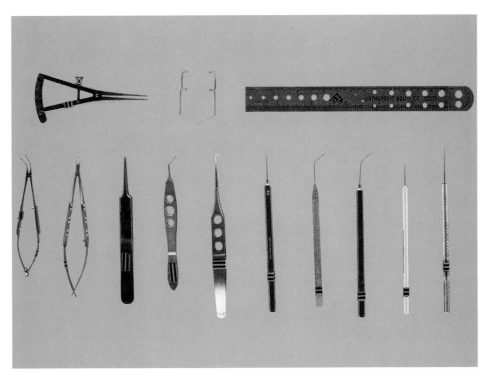

70-1 *Top, left to right,* 1 Castroviejo caliper; 1 Barraquer wire speculum; 1 metal ruler, small. *Bottom, left to right,* 1 Thornton IOL forceps; 1 Shephard intraocular lens forceps; 1 Simcoe nucleus removal forceps; 1 Kelman-McPherson forceps; 1 Clayman lens forceps; 1 Sinskey hook; 1 Hirschman serrated spatula; 1 Jaffe lens spatula; 1 Hirschman iris hook; 1 Graether collar button.

Eye Microinstruments

ADD CATARACT INSTRUMENTS AND BASIC EYE SET

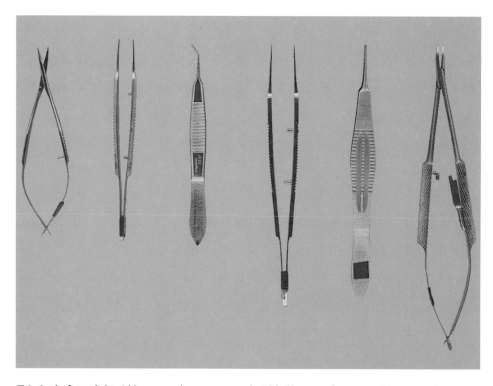

71-1 *Left to right,* 1 Vannas scissors, curved; 1 McPherson forceps without teeth, straight; 1 McPherson forceps without teeth, angled; 2 Castroviejo suturing forceps, 0.12 mm teeth (1 × 2); 1 Barraquer needle holder, extra delicate, tapered, curved, with lock.

72 Orbital Instruments

ADD BASIC EYE SET

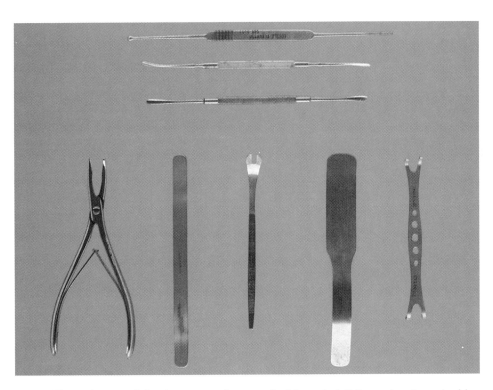

72-1 *Top to bottom,* 1 Cottle septum elevator, double ended; 2 Freer elevators, double ended. *Bottom, left to right,* 1 Belz lacrimal sac rongeur; 1 Dingman flexible retractor; 1 Schepens orbital retractor; 1 orbital retractor-elevator; 1 Converse alar retractor, double ended.

ADD BASIC EYE SET

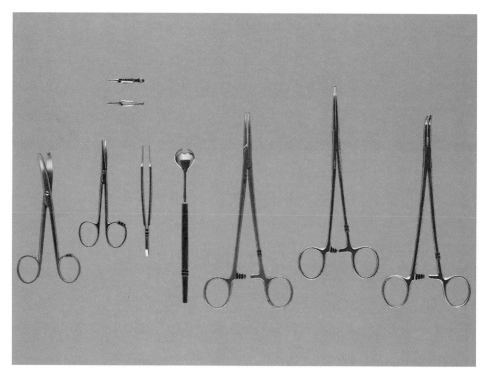

73-1 *Top,* 2 serrefines. *Bottom, left to right,* 1 enucleation scissors, sharp, curved; 1 Stevens tenotomy scissors; 1 Castroviejo suturing forceps with tying platforms, 0.5 mm teeth (1 × 2); 1 Schepens orbital retractor; 2 tonsil hemostatic forceps; 1 Westphal hemostatic forceps.

Corneal Transplant Instruments

ADD BASIC EYE SET

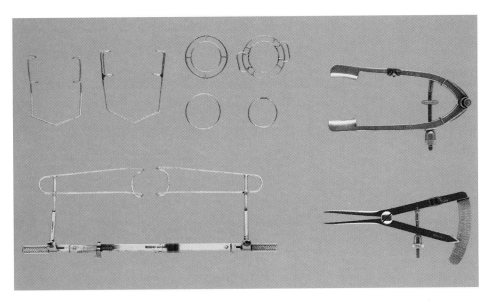

74-1 *Top, left to right,* 2 Barraquer wire speculums, opened wire, closed wire; 1 Flieringa fixation ring (double ring); 1 McNeil-Goldman scleral ring (with wings); 2 single-wire Flieringa fixation rings; 1 Lancaster speculum. *Bottom, left to right,* 1 Katena retractor; 1 Castroviejo caliper.

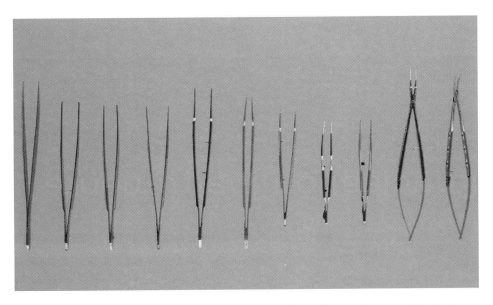

74-2 *Left to right,* 1 jeweler's forceps, straight; 1 O'Brien fixation forceps; 1 Elschnig fixation forceps; 1 serrated forceps, fine; 2 Castroviejo suturing forceps, 0.5 mm, 0.12 mm; 1 McPherson tying forceps, angled; 1 Colibri Troutman Barraquer forceps; 1 Polack double corneal forceps; 1 Maumenee corneal forceps; 1 Clayman lens forceps.

74-3 *Top, left to right,* 1 Sheets irrigating vectus, 27 gauge; 3 irrigating cannulas, 19, 23, and 27 gauge. *Bottom, left to right,* 1 Beaver knife handle, knurled, with insert; 1 corneal scleral marker; 1 Shepard iris hook; 1 Osher Y hook; 1 Sinskey iris and IOL hook; 1 Jaffe lens spatula; 1 Jameson muscle hook; 1 lens loop; 1 Paton spatula, double ended; 1 Castroviejo needle holder with lock, curved; 1 titanium needle holder with stop, no lock, curved; 1 Sinskey tying forceps, straight; 1 small-tipped needle holder without lock, curved.

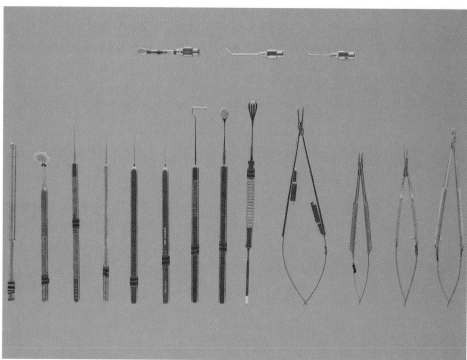

74-4 *Left to right,* 2 Halstead mosquito hemostatic forceps; 2 blunt scissors, straight; 2 Castroviejo corneal section scissors, left, right; 1 Vannas scissors, straight; 2 transplant microscissors, right, left; 1 Westcott tenotomy scissors.

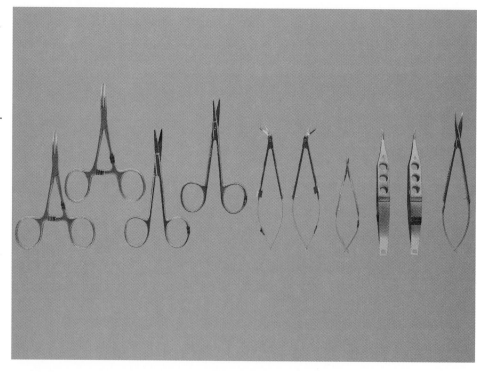

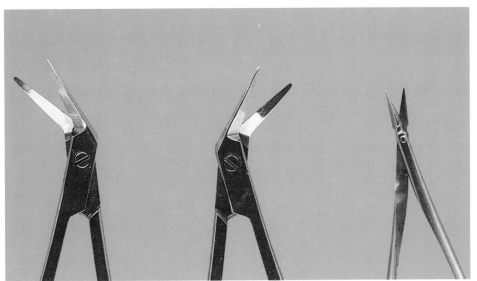

74-5 *Left to right,* Enlarged tips: Castroviejo corneal section scissors, left, right; Vannas scissors, straight.

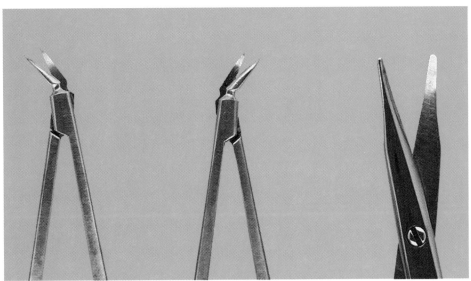

74-6 *Left to right,* Enlarged tips: 2 transplant microscissors, left, right; Westcott tenotomy scissors, blunt.

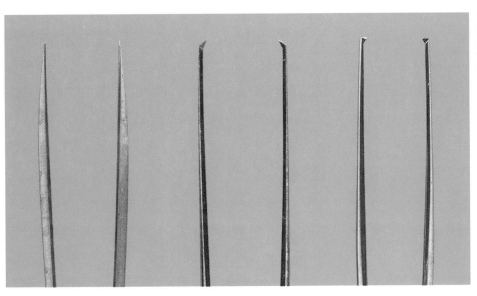

74-7 *Left to right,* Enlarged tips: 1 jeweler's forceps; 1 O'Brien fixation forceps; 1 Elschnig fixation forceps.

74-8 *Left to right,*
Enlarged tips: 2 Castroviejo suturing forceps, 0.5 mm, 0.12 mm, with teeth (1 × 2).

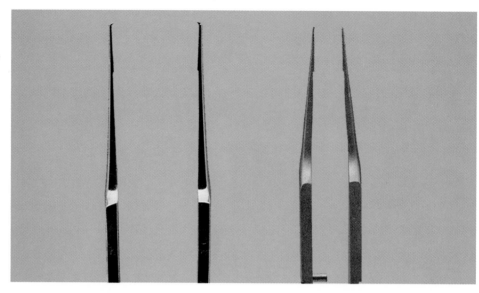

74-9 *Left to right,*
Enlarged tips: 1 McPherson tying forceps, angled; 1 Colibrí corneal utility forceps; 1 Polack double corneal forceps.

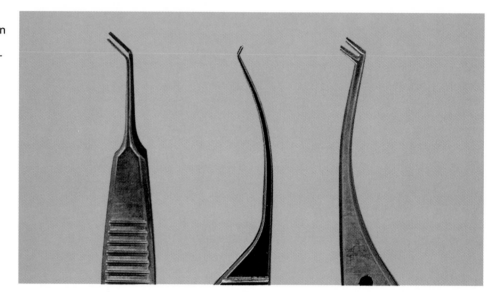

74-10 *Left to right,*
Enlarged tips: 1 Clayman lens-holding forceps; 1 Maumenee corneal forceps; 1 Sinskey tying forceps, straight.

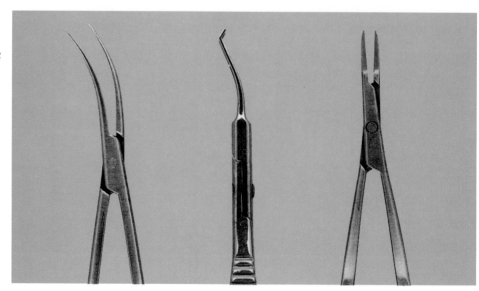

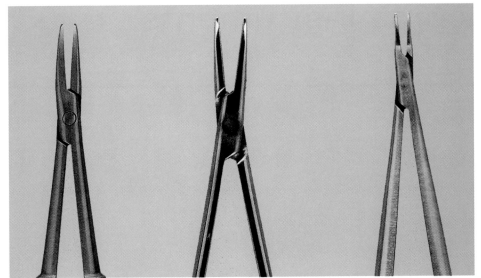

74-11 *Left to right,* Enlarged tips: 1 titanium needle holder, no lock; 1 Castroviejo needle holder; 1 small-tipped needle holder, curved.

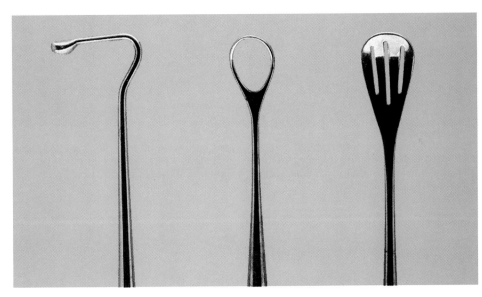

74-12 *Left to right,* Enlarged tips: 1 Jameson muscle hook; 1 lens loop; 1 Paton spatula, double ended.

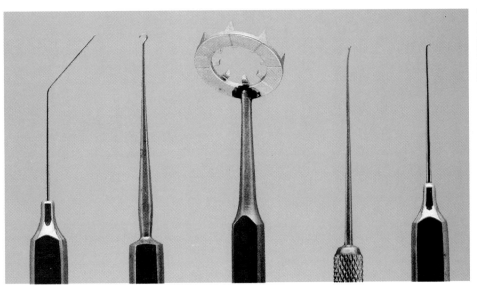

74-13 *Left to right,* Enlarged tips: 1 Jaffee lens spatula; 1 Shepard iris hook; 1 corneal scleral marker; 1 Osher Y hook; 1 Sinskey iris and IOL hook.

ADD BASIC EYE SET

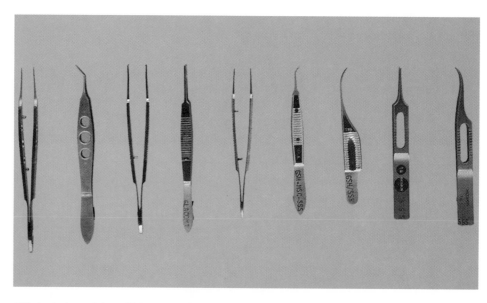

75-1 *Left to right,* 2 Kelman-McPherson tying forceps, straight, front view, angled, side view; 2 McCullough utility forceps, front view, side view; 1 McPherson tying forceps, straight; 1 McPherson tying forceps, curved; 1 Chandler (Gills) forceps; 2 Hoskins forceps, straight, curved.

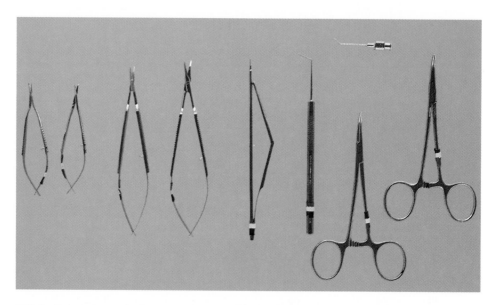

75-2 *Top, right,* 1 irrigation cannula, 19 gauge. *Bottom, left to right,* 2 Vannas scissors, straight, curved; 1 mini–Westcott corneal miniscissors, sharp; 1 Westcott tenotomy scissors, blunt; 1 Kelley decemet membrane punch; 1 Elschnig cyclodialysis spatula; 2 Halstead mosquito hemostatic forceps, curved.

76

Dacryocystorhinotomy

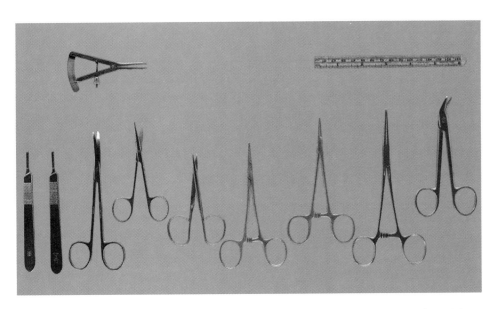

76-1 *Top, left to right,* 1 Castroviejo caliper; 1 metal ruler, 6 inch. *Bottom, left to right,* 2 Bard Parker knife handles, No. 3; 1 Metzenbaum scissors, 5 inch; 1 sharp/sharp iris scissors, 4 inch; 1 Stevens tenotomy scissors, curved; 2 Halstead mosquito hemostatic forceps, straight; 1 Halstead hemostatic forceps; 1 wire scissors.

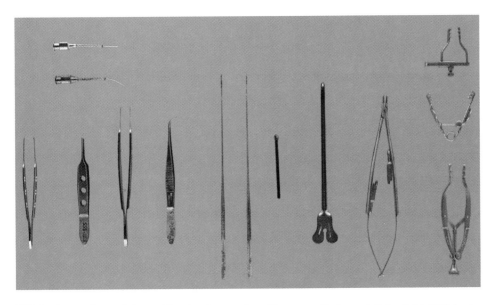

76-2 *Top, left,* 2 reinforced lacrimal cannulas, 23 gauge. *Bottom, left to right,* 2 Bishop-Harmon tissue forceps, front view, side view; 1 Castroviejo suturing forceps, 0.5 mm, front view; 1 iris forceps, 60-degree curve, side view; 2 metal cotton applicators; 1 round cutting bur, 1/8 × 2 3/4 inch; 1 grooved director; 1 Castroviejo needle holder with lock, straight. *Right, top to bottom,* 1 Goldstein lacrimal sac retractor; 1 Agricola lacrimal sac retractor; 1 Stevenson lacrimal sac retractor.

76-3 *Left to right,* 4 Freer elevators, double ended, 3 straight, 1 curved; 1 Cottle elevator, double ended; 1 Jameson muscle hook; 1 Burnisher dental tool; 1 Belz lacrimal rongeur; 2 Freer chisels, straight, curved; 1 mallet with lead-filled head, small.

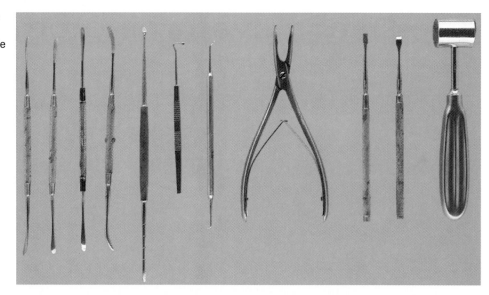

76-4 *Left to right,* Tips: 2 Freer elevators, double ended, straight, curved; 1 Cottle elevator, double ended; 1 Jameson muscle hook; 1 Burnisher dental tool; 2 Freer chisels, straight, curved.

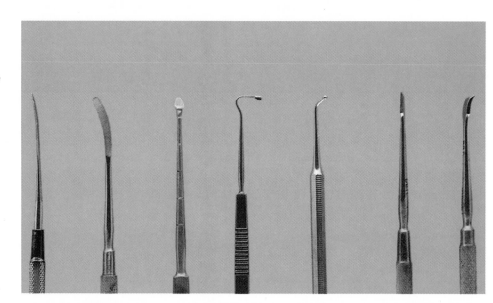

76-5 *Left, top to bottom,* 1 Ziegler lacrimal dilator, double ended, curved; 1 Heath punctal dilator; 1 infant lacrimal dilator. *Right, top to bottom,* 1 Castroviejo lacrimal dilator, double ended; 1 Wilder lacrimal dilator, single ended, straight. *Bottom, left to right,* 4 Bowman lacrimal probes, 2 of 0000-000, 2 of 00-0; 2 Jones punctal dilators with sharp tips, 1-2; 7 Bowman lacrimal probes, 2 of 1-2, 2 of 3-4, 2 of 5-6, 1 of 7-8.

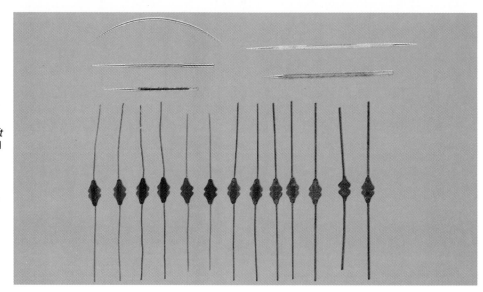

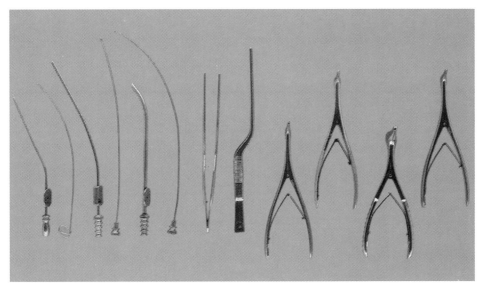

76-6 *Left to right,* 3 suction tubes with stylets: 1 Baron, 5 Fr; 1 Frazier, 7 Fr; 1 Adson, 11 Fr; 2 bayonet forceps, 6³/8 inch, 7¹/4 inch; 2 Cottle nasal speculums, 1 × ¹/2 inch; 1 Vienna nasal speculum, 2 × 1 inch; 1 Cottle nasal speculum, 1 × 1¹/4 inch.

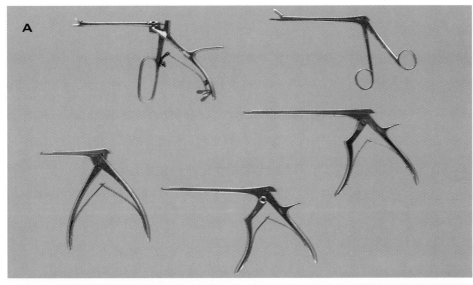

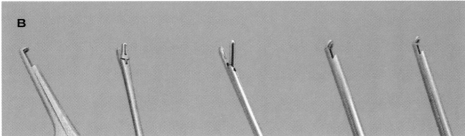

76-7 **A**, *Left, top to bottom,* 1 Miles nasal punch tip in universal handle; 1 Kerrison rongeur, 3¹/2 inch, 90-degree upbite. *Right, top to bottom,* 1 pituitary rongeur, straight, 5¹/2 inch; 1 Kerrison micro-rongeur, 3 mm, 40-degree upbite, 7 inch; 1 Kerrison rongeur, 6 inch, 40-degree upbite. **B**, *Left to right,* Tips: 1 Kerrison rongeur, 3¹/2 inch, 90-degree upbite; 1 Miles nasal punch tip; 1 pituitary rongeur, straight; 2 Kerrison rongeurs, 40-degree upbite, 1st 6 inch; 2nd micro-, 3 mm, 7 inch.

Basic Ear Set

77-1 *Top, left to right,* 2 paper drape clips; 2 Backhaus towel forceps, small. *Bottom, left to right,* 1 Bard Parker knife handle, No. 3; 2 Adson tissue forceps, without teeth, with teeth (1 × 2); 1 Brown Adson tissue forceps with teeth (7 × 7); 1 Sheehy ossicle-holding forceps; 1 strabismus scissors, curved; 2 Halstead mosquito hemostatic forceps, curved; 2 Crile hemostatic forceps; 1 Mayo dissecting scissors, straight; 1 Johnson needle holder.

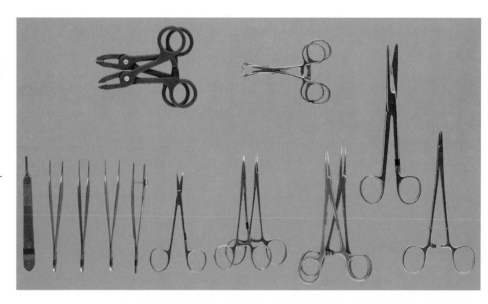

77-2 *Left, top to bottom,* 1 Weitlaner retractor, dull prongs, angled; 3 Baron ear suction tubes with finger valve control, 3, 5, and 7 Fr, and 1 stylet. *Right, top to bottom,* 9 Richard ear speculums, assorted sizes, 4 to 8 mm, one side view. *Bottom, left to right,* 1 Cottle elevator, double ended; 1 Lempert elevator (converse periosteal); 2 Johnson skin hooks; 2 Senn-Kanavel retractors, side view, front view; 1 House Teflon block; 1 House Gelfoam press or Sheehy fascia press; 2 metal medicine cups, 2 oz.

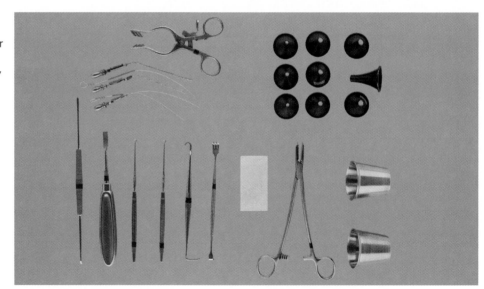

Delicate Ear Instruments

ADD BASIC EAR SET

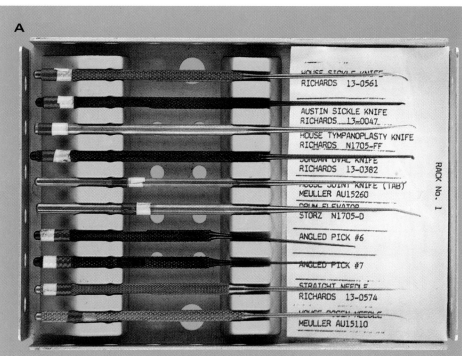

78-1 **A,** Rack No. 1 of delicate ear instruments with labels. **B,** *Left to right,* Tips of delicate ear instruments: House sickle knife; Austin sickle knife; House tympanoplasty knife. **C,** *Left to right,* Tips of delicate ear instruments: Jordan oval knife; House joint knife; drum elevator; angled pick, No. 6; angled pick, No. 7; straight needle; House Rosen needle.

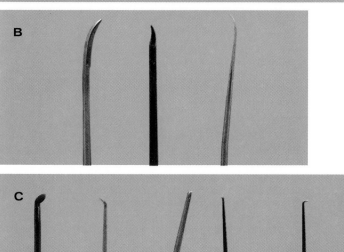

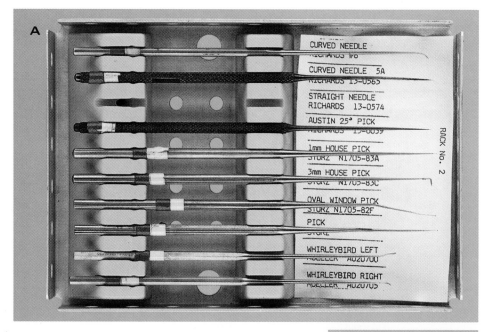

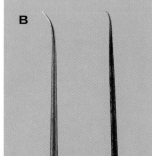

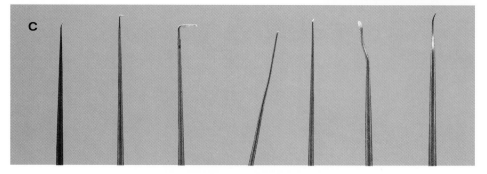

78-2 **A,** Rack No. 2 of delicate ear instruments with labels. **B,** *Left to right,* Tips of delicate ear instruments: 2 curved needles, large curve, small curve. **C,** *Left to right,* Tips of delicate ear instruments: straight needle; Austin 25-degree pick; House pick, 1 mm; House pick, 3 mm; oval window pick; 2 Whirleybird, left, right.

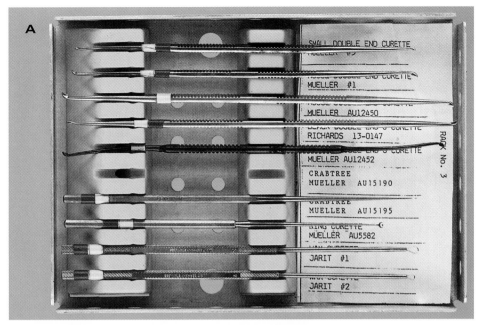

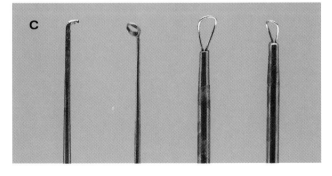

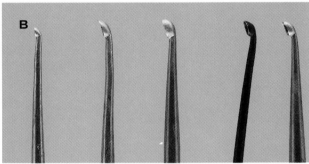

78-3 A, Rack No. 3 of delicate ear instruments with labels. **B,** *Left to right,* Tips of delicate ear instruments: small double-end curette No. 3; House double-end curette No. 1; House double-end curette; Black double-end J curette; House double-end J curette. **C,** *Left to right,* Tips of delicate ear instruments: Crabtree; ring curette; wax curette, No. 1; wax curette, No. 2.

78-4 A, Rack No. 4 of delicate ear instruments with labels. **B**, *Left to right,* Tips of delicate ear instruments: measuring rod; House measuring rod, 4 mm; House measuring rod, 4.5 mm; House measuring rod. **C**, *Left to right,* Tips of delicate ear instruments: measuring rod; Derlacki; angled pick. **D**, *Left to right,* Tips of delicate ear instruments: delicate hook, No. 14; Buckingham footplate hand drill; Rosen knife.

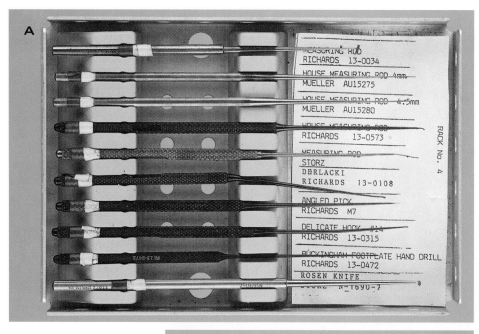

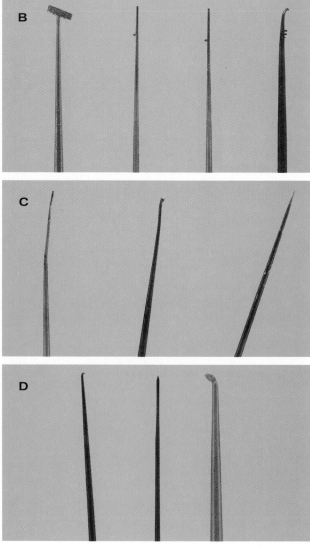

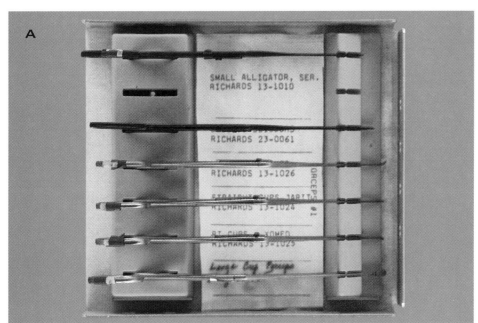

A

SMALL ALLIGATOR, SER.
RICHARDS 13-1010

RICHARDS 23-0061

RICHARDS 13-1026

RICHARDS 13-1024

RICHARDS 13-1025

78-5 A, Tray No. 1 delicate ear forceps with labels. **B**, Delicate ear forceps out of tray. **C**, *Left to right*, Tips of delicate ear forceps: small alligator, serrated; Belucci scissors; left-cup forceps. **D**, *Left to right*, Tips of delicate ear forceps: straight-cup forceps; right-cup forceps; large-cup forceps.

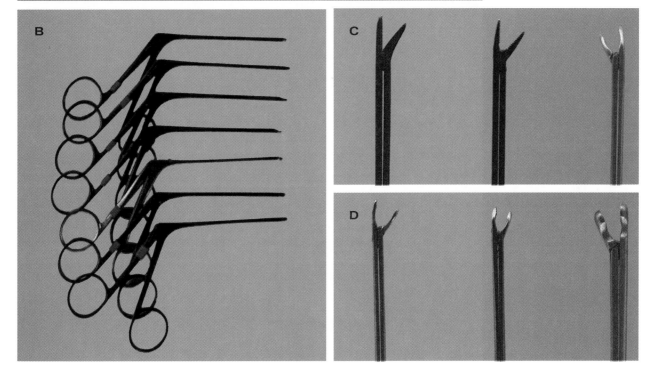

B

C

D

78-6 A, Tray No. 2 delicate ear forceps with labels. **B,** *Left to right,* Tips of delicate ear forceps: large crimper, small crimper; malleus nipper.

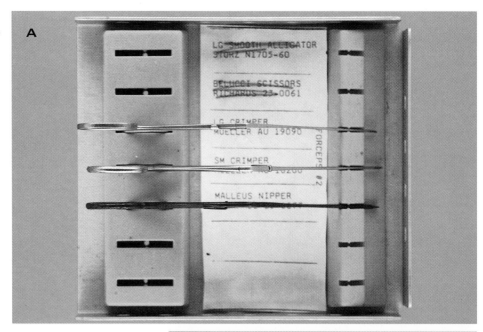

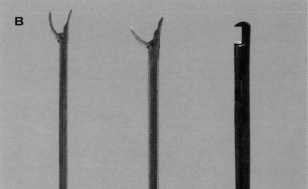

78-7 Blunt needles attached to tubing for suction tips, assorted sizes, 15 gauge to 24 gauge.

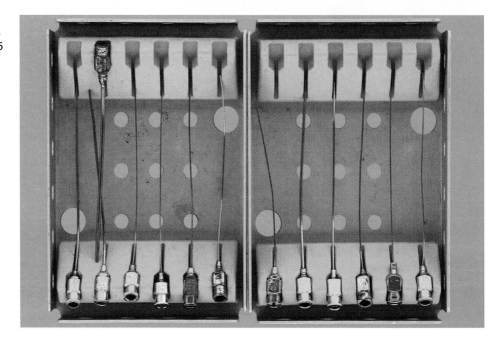

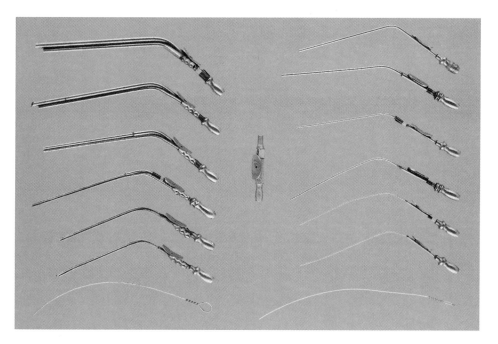

78-8 *Left to right,* 6 House suction/irrigators with finger valve control and 1 stylet; 1 metal suction connector; 6 Baron ear suction tubes with finger valve control and 1 stylet.

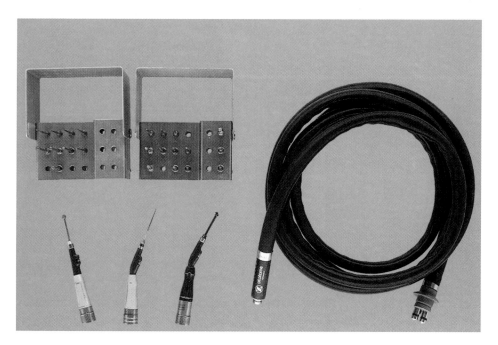

78-9 Ototome drill with bits and power cord: straight high-speed handpiece; angled high-speed handpiece; angled low-speed handpiece; diamond burs; cutting burs; air microburs.

79

Myringotomy Set

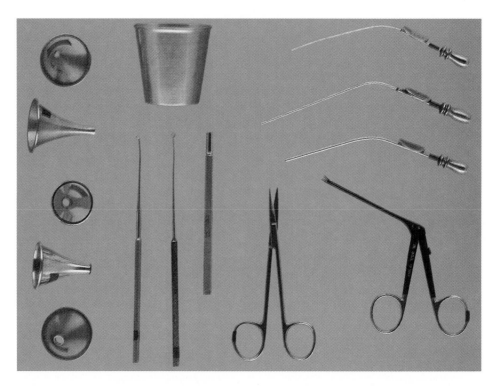

79-1 *Left, top to bottom,* 5 Bouchern ear speculums, assorted sizes. *Top, left to right,* 1 metal medicine cup, 8 oz; 3 Frazier suction tubes. *Bottom, left to right,* 2 ear curettes, small, large; 1 myringotomy knife in folding handle with straight Royce blade; 1 iris scissors, straight; 1 alligator forceps, straight.

80

Nasal Set

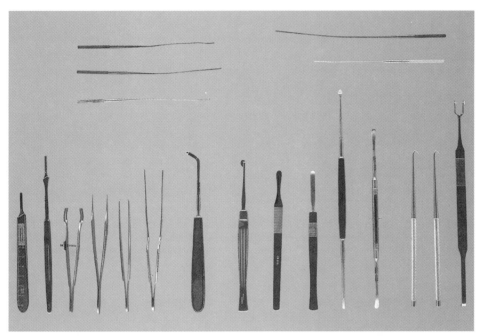

80-1 *Top,* 5 Ludwig wire applicators. *Bottom, left to right,* 2 Bard Parker knife handles, No. 3, No. 7; 1 Cottle columella forceps; 1 Brown Adson tissue forceps with teeth (7 × 7); 1 Beasley Babcock tissue forceps; 1 Jansen thumb forceps, bayonet shaft, serrated tips; 1 Joseph button end knife, curved; 1 Freer septum knife; 1 Cottle nasal knife; 1 McKenty elevator; 1 Cottle septum elevator; 1 Freer elevator; 2 Joseph skin hooks; 1 Cottle knife guide and retractor.

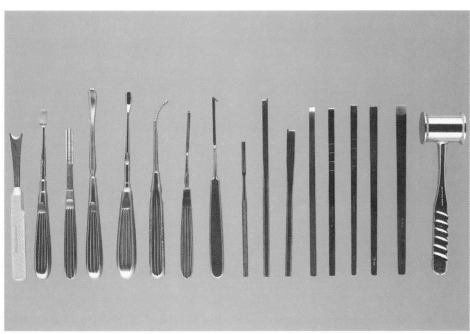

80-2 *Left to right,* 1 Bauer rocking chisel; 1 Lewis rasp; 1 Maltz rasp; 2 Aufricht rasps, large, small; 1 Wiener antrum rasp; 2 Ballenger swivel knives; 1 Ballenger chisel, 4 mm; 2 Converse guarded osteotomes; 1 Cottle osteotome, round corners, curved, 6 mm; 4 Cottle osteotomes, straight, 4, 7, 9, and 12 mm; 1 mallet, lead-filled head.

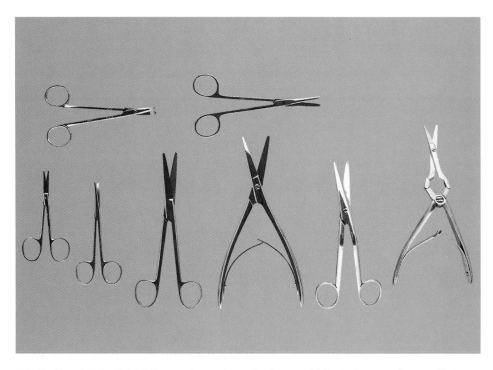

80-3 *Top, left to right,* 1 Fomon lower lateral scissors; 1 Metzenbaum scissors. *Bottom, left to right,* 2 Metzenbaum scissors, 4 inch, straight, curved; 1 Mayo dissecting scissors, straight; 1 Cottle spring scissors; 1 Cottle dorsal angular scissors; 1 Becker septum scissors.

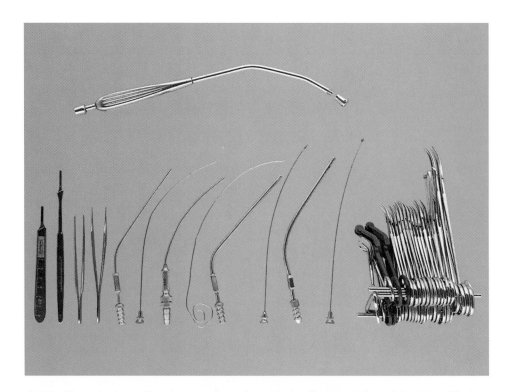

80-4 *Top,* 1 Andrews Pynchon suction tube with tip. *Bottom, left to right,* 2 Bard Parker knife handles, No. 3, No. 7; 1 Beasley Babcock tissue forceps; 1 Brown Adson tissue forceps with teeth (7 × 7); 4 Frazier suction tubes with stylets, 2 of 7 Fr, 2 of 12 Fr; 2 Backhaus towel forceps, small; 2 paper drape clips; 12 Halstead mosquito hemostatic forceps, curved; 2 Allis tissue forceps; 2 tonsil hemostatic forceps; 1 Johnson needle holder.

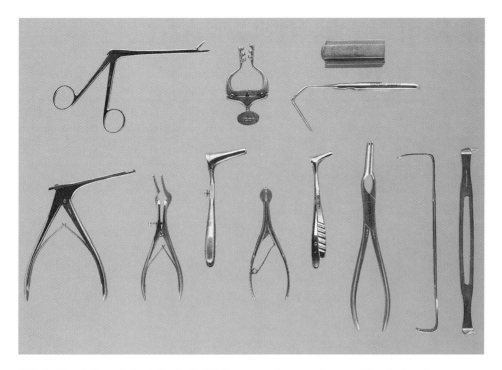

80-5 *Top, left to right,* 1 Ferris-Smith fragment forceps; 1 mastoid articulated retractor; 1 Cottle bone crusher, closed; 1 Aufricht retractor. *Bottom, left to right,* 1 Kerrison rongeur, upbite; 2 Killian nasal speculums: 2 inch, front view; 3 inch, side view; 2 Vienna nasal speculums: 1³/₈ inch, front view; 1¹/₈ inch, side view; 1 Asch septum forceps; 2 Army Navy retractors, side view, front view.

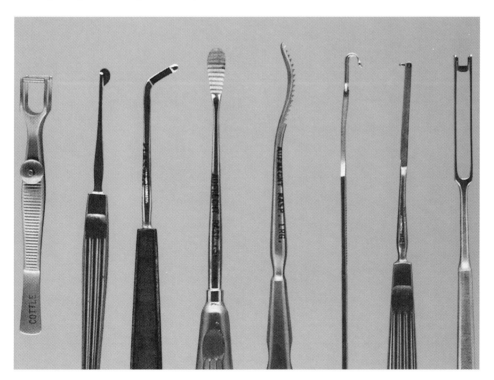

80-6 *Left to right,* Tips: 1 Cottle columella forceps; 1 Freer septum knife; 1 Joseph button end knife; 2 Aufricht rasps, small, front view; large, side view; 1 Cottle knife guide and retractor, side view; 2 Ballenger swivel knives, side view, front view.

Nasal Polyp Instruments

ADD NASAL SET

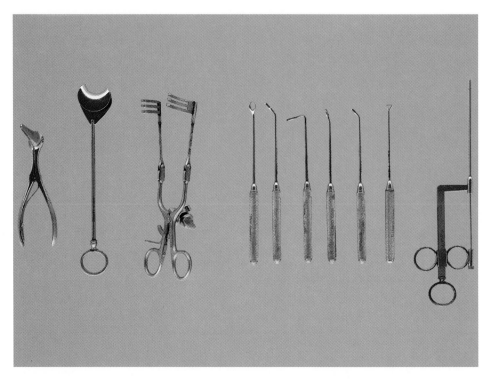

81-1 *Left to right,* 1 Killian nasal speculum, 3 inch; 1 Druck-Levine antrum retractor with blade (1st); 6 Coakley antrum curettes: assorted sizes, No. 1 to 6; 1 Bruening nasal snare, bayonet (disposable wire).

82 Nasal Reduction Instruments

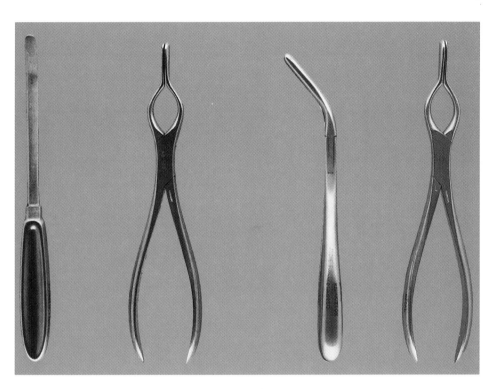

82-1 *Left to right,* 1 Gillies elevator; 3 Asche forceps, assorted angles.

Tonsil and Adenoid Set

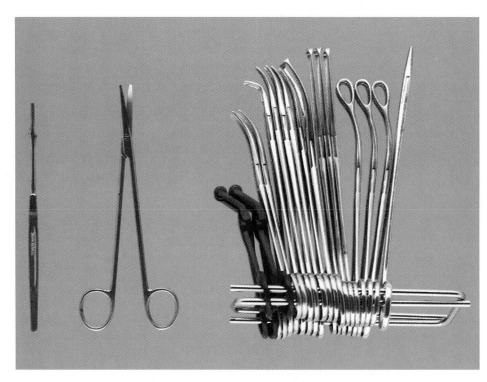

83-1 *Left to right,* 1 Bard Parker knife handle, No. 7; 1 Metzenbaum scissors, 7 inch; 2 paper drape clips; 2 Crile hemostatic forceps, 6½ inch; 1 Westphal hemostatic forceps; 4 tonsil hemostatic forceps; 1 Allis tissue forceps, long, curved; 3 Allis tissue forceps, long; 3 Ballenger sponge forceps, curved; 1 Crile Wood needle holder, 8 inch.

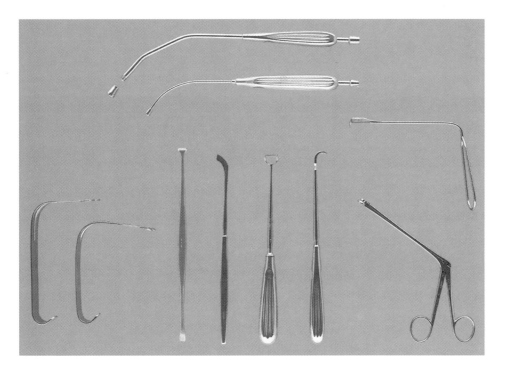

83-2 *Top to bottom,* 1 Andrews Pynchon suction tube with tip; 1 adenoid suction tube, tip connected. *Bottom, left to right,* 2 Wieder tongue depressors; 1 Hurd tonsil dissector and pillar retractor; 1 Fisher tonsil knife and dissector; 2 LaForce adenotomes: small, front view; large, side view. *Top middle, right,* 1 Lothrop uvula retractor. *Bottom right,* 1 Meltzer adenoid punch, round, with basket.

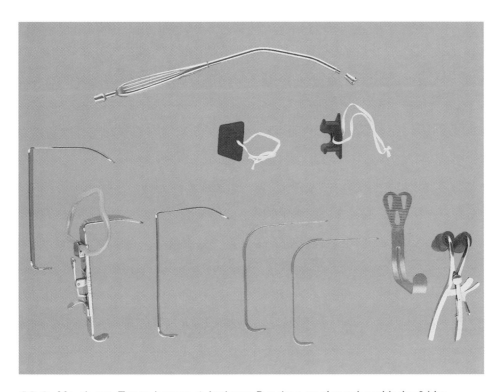

83-3 Mouth set. *Top to bottom,* 1 Andrews Pynchon suction tube with tip; 2 bite blocks, child, adult. *Left to right,* 1 McIvor mouth gag frame with blade and 2 other blades; 3 Weider tongue depressors, 2 side views, 1 front view; 1 side mouth gag.

Unit Nine

ORTHOPEDIC SURGERY

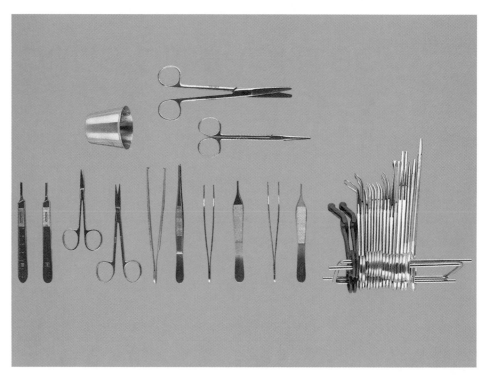

84-1 *Top, left to right,* 1 metal medicine cup, 2 oz; 1 Mayo dissecting scissors, straight; 1 Metzenbaum scissors, 5 inch. *Bottom, left to right,* 2 Bard Parker knife handles, No. 3; 2 plastic scissors: straight, sharp; curved, sharp; 2 thumb tissue forceps with teeth (1 × 2), front view, side view; 2 Adson tissue forceps with teeth (1 × 2), front view, side view; 2 Brown Adson tissue forceps with teeth (7 × 7), front view, side view; 2 paper drape clips; 2 Backhaus towel forceps; 6 Halstead mosquito hemostatic forceps, curved; 2 Crile hemostatic forceps, curved, 5½ inch; 2 Allis tissue forceps; 2 Ochsner hemostatic forceps; 3 Crile Wood needle holders, 2 of 6 inch, 1 of 7 inch.

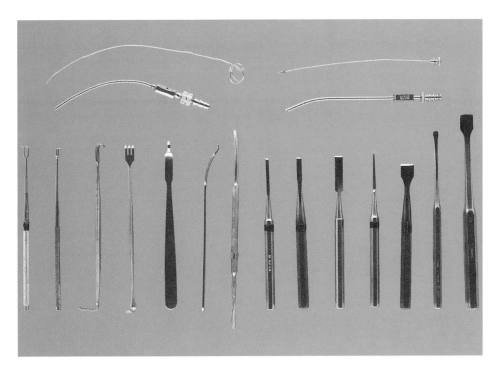

84-2 *Top,* 2 Adson suction tubes, finger valve controls, stylets, 9 Fr, 11 Fr. *Bottom, left to right,* 2 Joseph skin hooks, double prong, front view, side view; 2 Miller-Senn retractors, side view, front view; 2 Hohman retractors, mini-, front view, side view; 1 Freer elevator; 5 Hoke chisels, assorted sizes; 2 Key periosteal elevators, 1/4 inch, 1/2 inch.

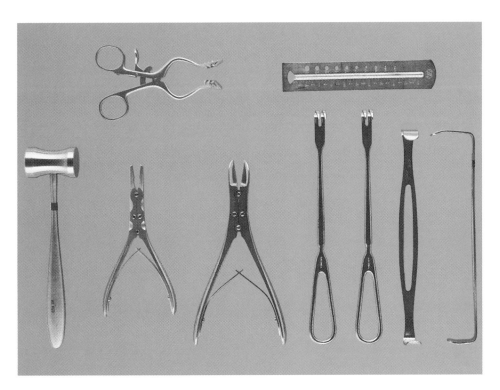

84-3 *Top, left to right,* 1 Weitlaner retractor, baby, curved; 1 metal ruler, 6 inch. *Bottom, left to right,* 1 mallet; 1 Ruskin rongeur, double action; 1 Ruskin-Liston bone-cutting forceps; 2 Volkmann retractors, 2 pronged, sharp; 2 Army Navy retractors, front view, side view.

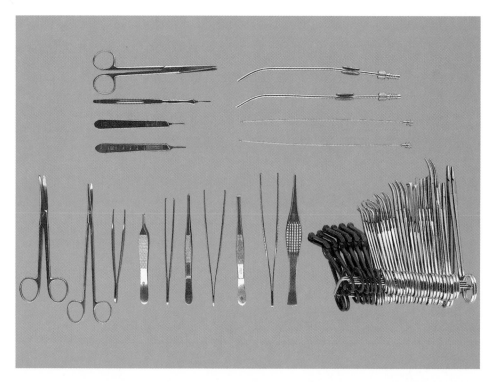

85-1 *Left, top to bottom,* 1 Mayo dissecting scissors, straight; 3 Bard Parker knife handles, 1 No. 7, 2 No. 3. *Top, right,* 2 Adson suction tubes, curved, finger valve controls, and with stylets. *Bottom, left to right,* 1 Mayo dissecting scissors, curved; 1 Metzenbaum scissors, 7 inch; 2 Adson tissue forceps with teeth (1 × 2), front view, side view; 2 thumb tissue forceps with teeth (1 × 2), front view, side view; 2 thumb tissue forceps with multiteeth (4 × 5), front view, side view; 2 Ferris-Smith tissue forceps, front view, side view; 6 paper drape clips; 4 Halstead mosquito hemostatic forceps, curved; 2 Backhaus towel forceps; 4 Crile hemostatic forceps, 5¹/₂ inch; 4 Crile hemostatic forceps, 6¹/₂ inch; 2 Allis tissue forceps; 4 Ochsner hemostatic forceps, short; 2 tonsil hemostatic forceps; 4 Crile Wood needle holders, 2 of 6 inch, 2 of 7 inch.

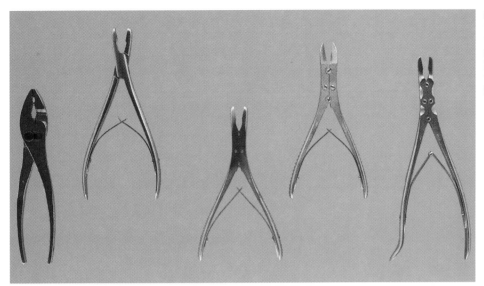

85-2 *Left to right,* 1 pliers; 1 Luer bone rongeur; 1 Adson rongeur, double action; 1 Ruskin-Liston bone-cutting forceps; 1 Smith-Peterson laminectomy rongeur.

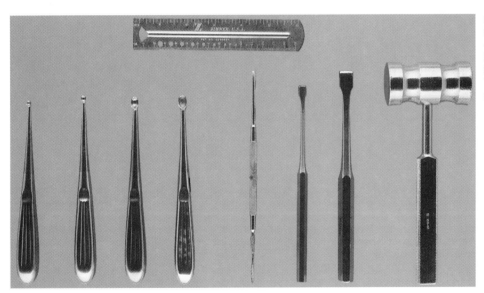

85-3 *Top,* 1 metal ruler, 6 inch. *Bottom, left to right,* 4 Spratt curettes, No. 2 to No. 5; 1 Freer elevator; 2 Key periosteal elevators, $1/4$ inch, $1/2$ inch; 1 metal mallet.

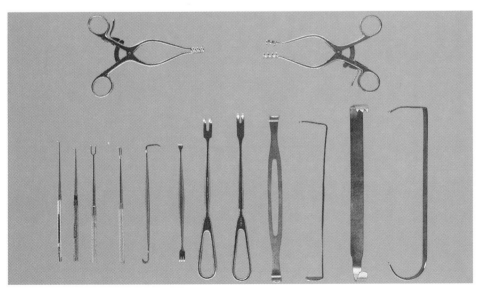

85-4 *Top,* 2 Weitlaner retractors, sharp pronged, medium. *Bottom, left to right,* 4 Joseph skin hooks: 2 single pronged, side view; 2 double pronged, front view, side view; 2 Miller-Senn retractors, side view, front view; 2 Volkmann retractors, 2 pronged, sharp; 2 Army Navy retractors, front view, side view; 2 Hibbs laminectomy retractors, narrow, front view, side view.

86

Shoulder Instruments

ADD SOFT TISSUE SET

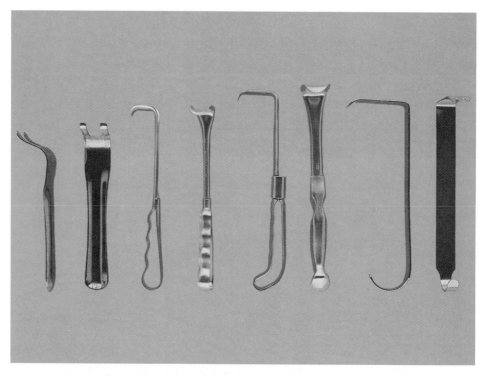

86-1 *Left to right,* 2 humeral head retractors, side view, front view; 4 Richardson retractors, 2 small, 2 medium, side view, front view; 2 Hibbs laminectomy retractors, side view, front view.

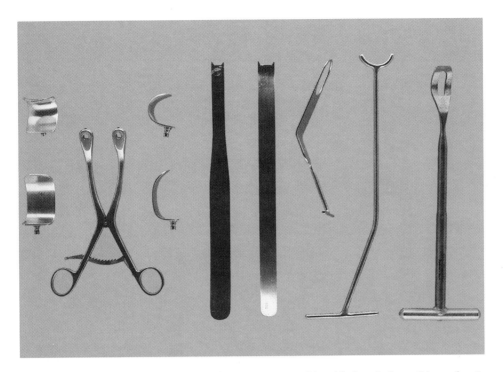

86-2 *Left to right,* 1 Gelnoid self-retaining retractor with 4 blades, 2 short, 2 long, front view, side view; 2 Gelnoid (Batman) retractors, narrow, medium; 1 shoulder retractor, angled, short; 1 Bankhardt shoulder retractor; 1 shoulder retractor, angled, long.

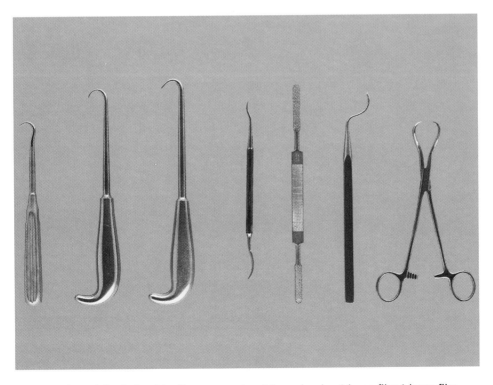

86-3 *Left to right,* 1 shoulder ligature carrier; 2 bone hooks; 1 bone file; 1 bone file; 1 Gelnoid punch; 1 Joplin bone forceps.

Power Drills and Saws

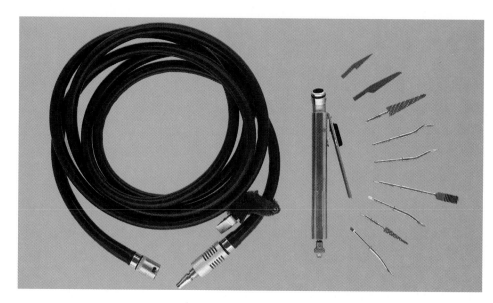

87-1   Reciprocating microsaw: power cord, saw handle, assorted blades.

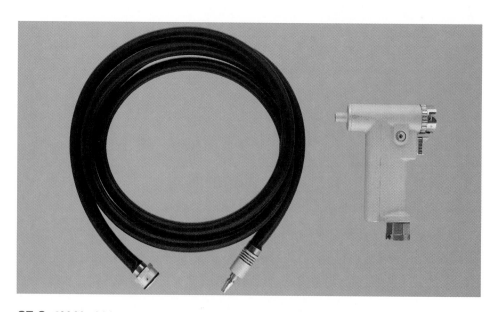

87-2   3M Maxidriver: power cord, driver.

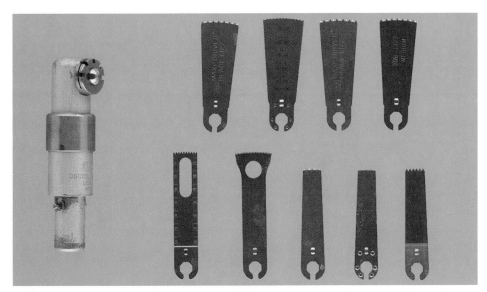

87-3 Oscillating saw: handle, assorted blades.

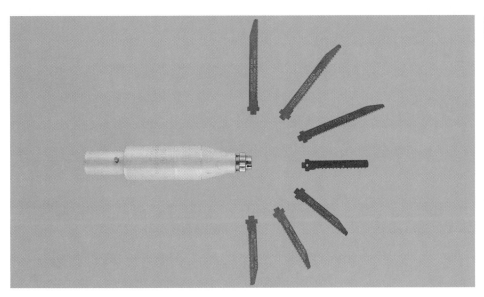

87-4 Reciprocating saw: handle, assorted blades.

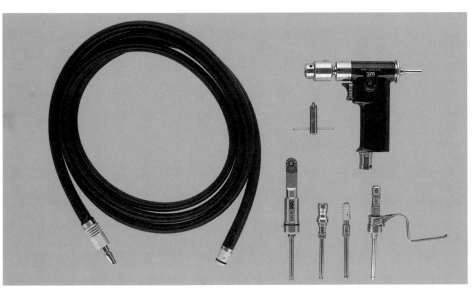

87-5 Maxidriver: power cord, driver, chuck, assorted blades.

88

Minor Joint Replacement Set

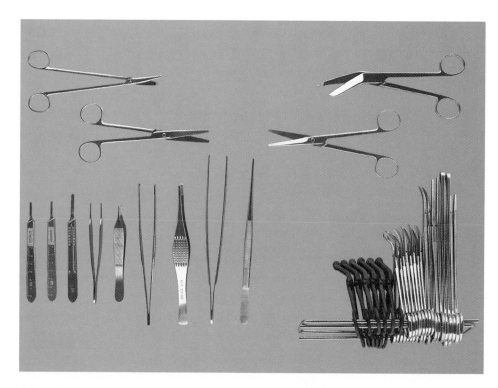

88-1 *Top to bottom, left to right,* 1 Metzenbaum scissors, 7 inch; 1 Mayo dissecting scissors, straight; 1 bandage scissors, 8 inch; 1 Mayo dissecting scissors, curved. *Bottom, left to right,* 3 Bard Parker knife handles, 2 No. 3, 1 No. 4; 2 Adson tissue forceps with teeth (1 × 2), front view, side view; 2 Ferris-Smith tissue forceps, front view, side view; 2 Cushing tissue forceps with teeth (1 × 2), 8 inch, front view, side view; 6 paper drape clips; 2 Backhaus towel forceps; 6 Crile hemostatic forceps, 5½ inch; 2 tonsil hemostatic forceps; 2 Ochsner hemostatic forceps, long; 2 Allis tissue forceps, long; 2 Crile Wood needle holders, 7 inch.

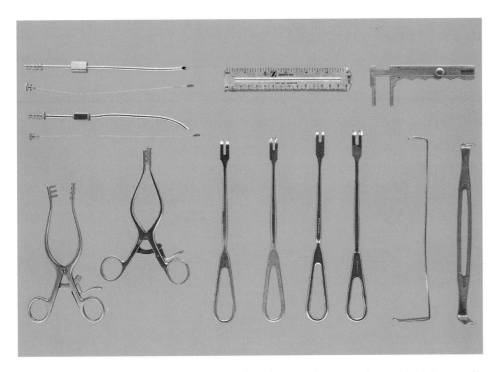

88-2 *Top, left to right,* 2 Adson suction tubes, finger valve control, 1 straight, 1 curved, with stylets; 1 metal ruler, 6 inch; 1 caliper, inside/outside. *Bottom, left to right,* 2 Weitlaner retractors, sharp, medium; 4 Volkmann retractors, 2 pronged: 2 sharp, 2 dull; 2 Army Navy retractors, side view, front view.

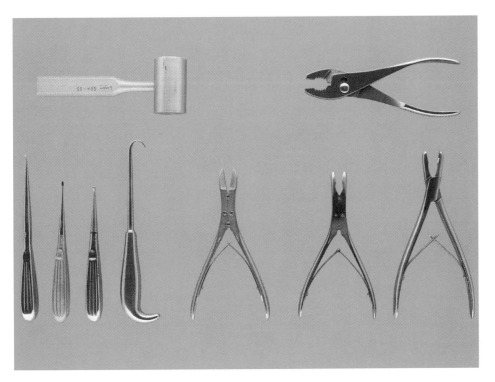

88-3 *Top, left to right,* 1 metal mallet; 1 pliers. *Bottom, left to right,* 3 Spratt curettes: long curved, 2-0, 3-0; 1 Ruskin-Liston bone-cutting forceps; 1 Adson rongeur, double-action; 1 Luer bone rongeur.

ADD MINOR JOINT REPLACEMENT SET. (These instruments were provided by Zimmer-Pasion Inc., Beaverton, OR.)

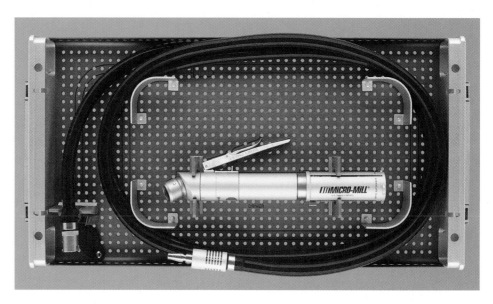

89-1 Micro–mill driver and attachments.

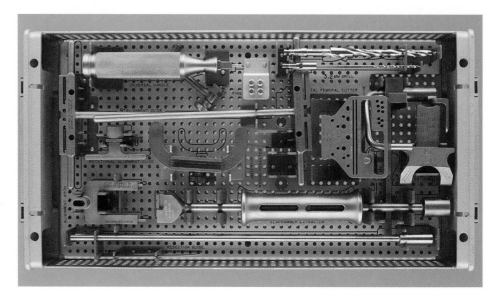

89-2 Intramedullar (IM) femoral alignment/resection instruments.

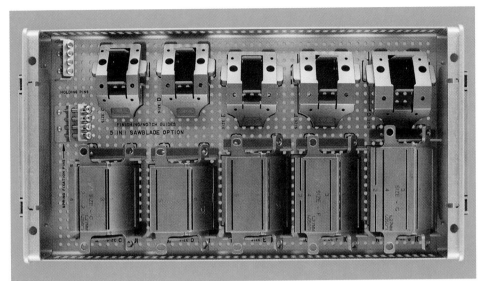

89-3 Femoral resection/finishing (5 in 1) instruments.

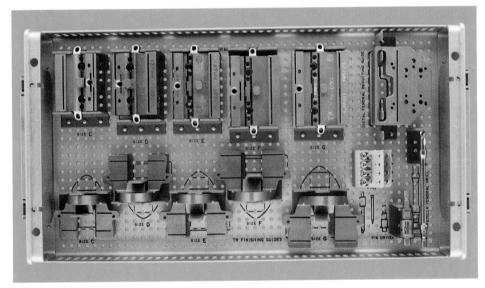

89-4 IM femoral finishing instruments.

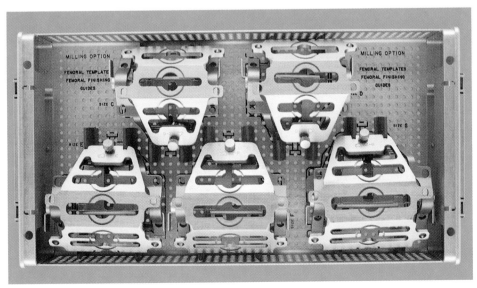

89-5 Femoral resection/finishing milling instruments.

89-6 Femoral sizing/alignment instruments.

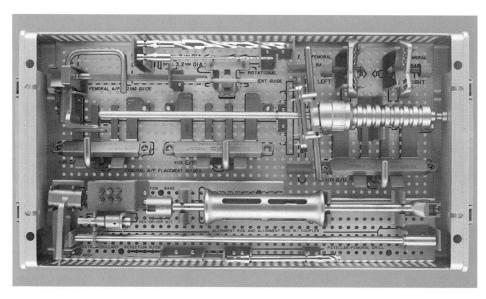

89-7 Cruciate retaining (CR) provisionals.

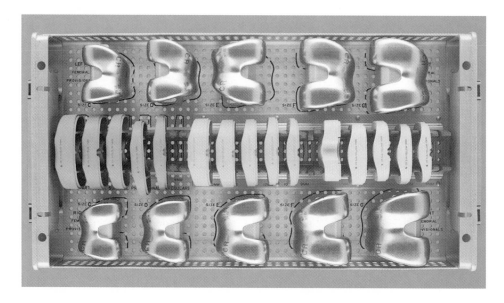

89-8 IM tibial alignment/finishing instruments.

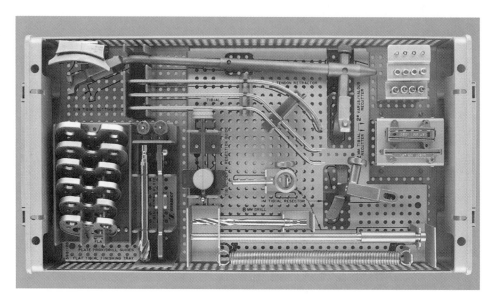

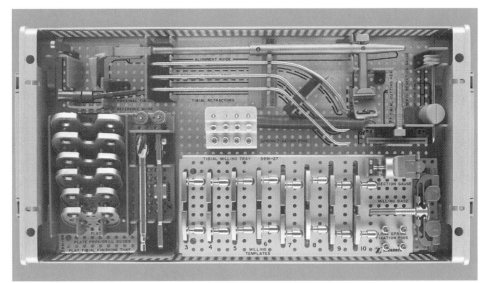

89-9 Tibial alignment/resection instruments.

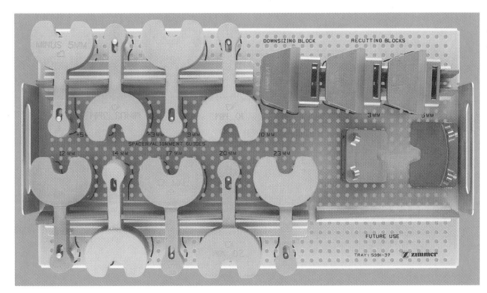

89-10 Patellar/spacer guide instruments (1st tray): spacer-alignment guides, recutting blocks.

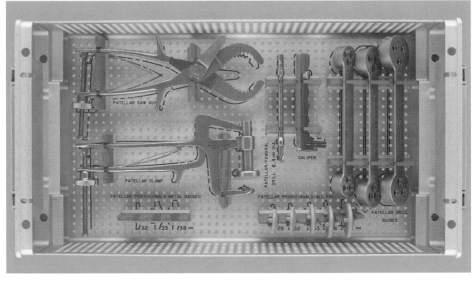

89-11 Patellar/spacer guide instruments (2nd tray).

89-12 Tibial femoral implant instruments (1st tray).

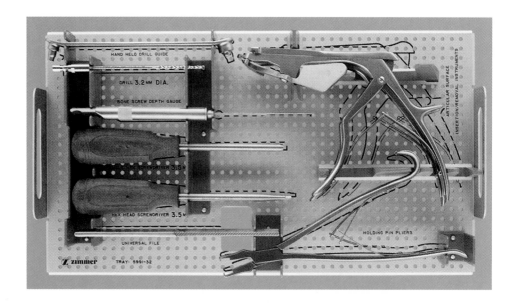

89-13 Tibial femoral implant instruments (2nd tray).

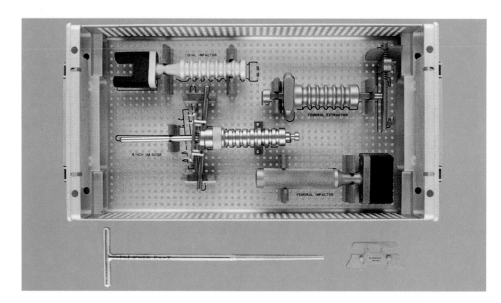

89-14 Alvarado knee support.

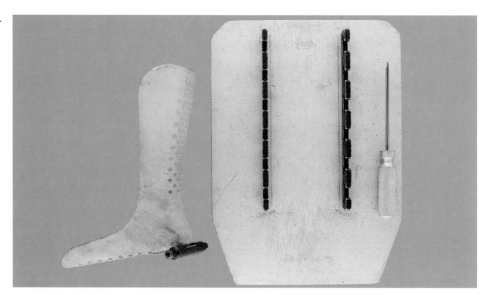

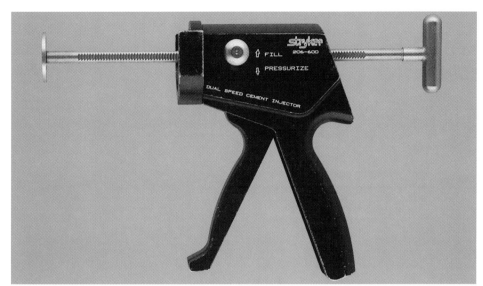

89-15 Stryker cement gun.

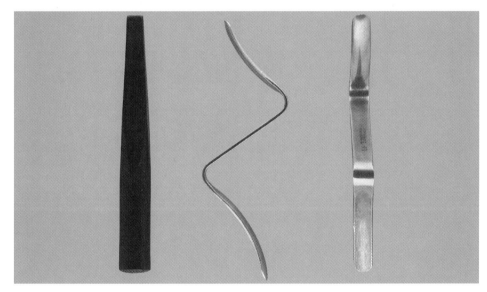

89-16 *Left to right,* 1 impactor; 2 Doane retractors, side view, front view.

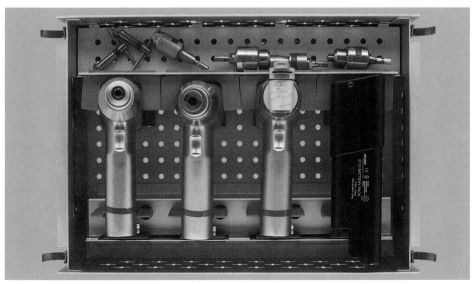

89-17 Stryker battery-powered drills in sterilizing tray.

89-18 *Top, left to right,* Stryker battery-powered drills: drill, adapter, chuck key, sagittal saw. *Bottom, left to right,* Adapter, reamer, battery pack.

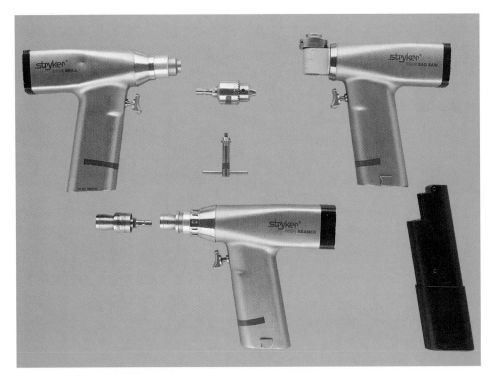

90

Total Knee Prosthesis

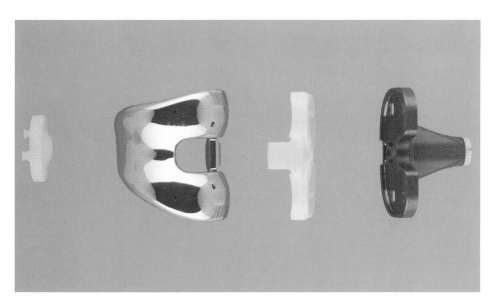

90-1 Nex Gen system. *Left to right,* 1 patella button; 1 femoral component; 1 articulating surface; 1 stem-tibial base plate.

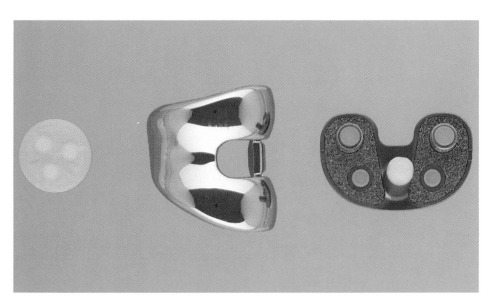

90-2 Nex Gen system. *Left to right,* 1 patella button; 1 femoral component; 1 porous stem–tibial base plate.

91

Open Reduction Hip Set

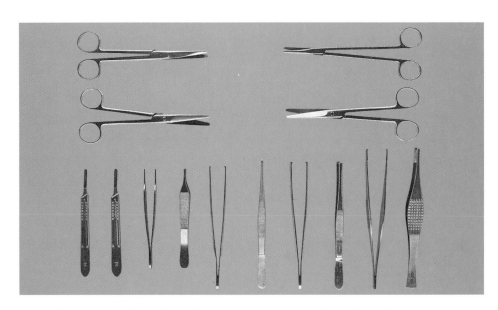

91-1 *Top, left to right,* 2 Mayo dissecting scissors, straight; 1 Metzenbaum scissors, 7 inch; 1 Mayo dissecting scissors, curved. *Bottom, left to right,* 2 Bard Parker knife handles, No. 4; 2 Adson tissue forceps with teeth (1 × 2), front view, side view; 2 thumb tissue forceps with teeth (1 × 2), front view, side view; 2 thumb tissue forceps with multi-teeth (4 × 5), front view, side view; 2 Ferris-Smith tissue forceps, front view, side view.

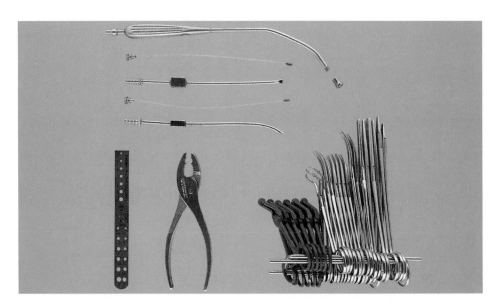

91-2 *Top to bottom,* 1 Yankauer suction tube with tip; 2 Adson suction tubes with finger valve controls, stylets, large. *Bottom, left to right,* 1 metal ruler, 6 inch; 1 pliers; 6 paper drape clips; 2 Backhaus towel forceps; 6 Crile hemostatic forceps, 6½ inch; 2 tonsil hemostatic forceps; 4 Ochsner hemostatic forceps, 8 inch; 2 Crile Wood needle holders, 8 inch.

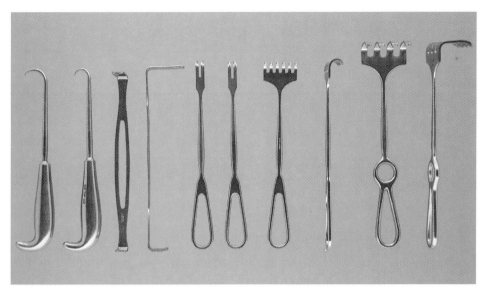

91-3 *Left to right,* 2 bone hooks; 2 Army Navy retractors, front view, side view; 4 Volkmann retractors: 2 with 2 pronged, sharp; 2 with 4 pronged, sharp, front view, side view; 2 Israel retractors, front view, side view.

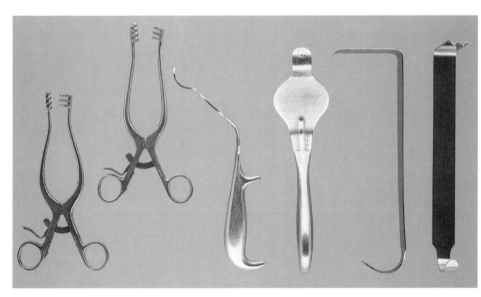

91-4 *Left to right,* 2 Weitlaner retractors, medium, sharp; 2 Bennett bone elevators and retractors, side view, front view; 2 Hibbs laminectomy retractors, medium, side view, front view.

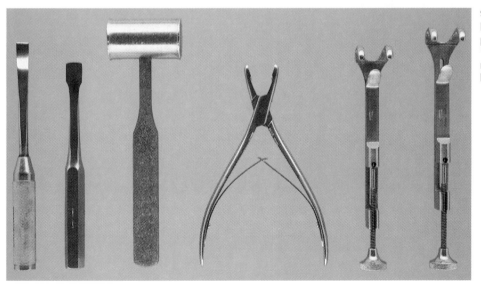

91-5 Left to right, 1 Scott-McCracken elevator; 1 Key periosteal elevator, 3/4 inch; 1 metal mallet; 1 Luer bone rongeur; 2 Lowman bone-holding clamps, front view.

92

Basic Total Hip Set

92-1 *Top,* 2 Volkmann retractors, 2 pronged, sharp. *Bottom, left to right,* 2 Bard-Parker knife handles, No. 4; 2 Adson tissue forceps with teeth (1 × 2), front view, side view; 1 thumb tissue forceps with teeth (1 × 2); 2 Ferris-Smith tissue forceps, front view, side view; 2 Mayo dissecting scissors, curved, straight; 4 paper drape clips; 2 Backhaus towel forceps; 2 Crile hemostatic forceps, 6½ inch; 2 tonsil hemostatic forceps; 1 Mayo Pean hemostatic forceps; 2 Ochsner hemostatic forceps; 1 Foerster sponge forceps; 2 Crile Wood needle holders, 8 inch.

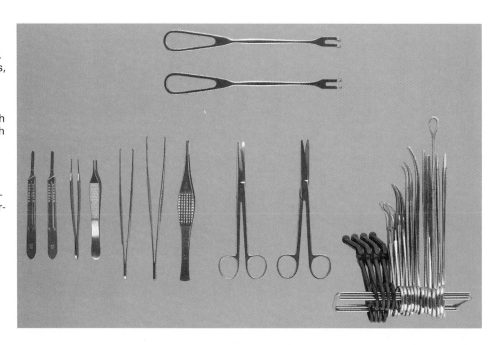

92-2 *Top, left to right,* 2 Yankauer suction tubes with tips; 2 Volkmann retractors, 6 pronged, sharp. *Bottom, left to right,* 1 Bard Parker knife handle, No. 4, long; 1 Russian tissue forceps, long; 1 Mayo dissecting scissors, curved, long; 1 bandage scissors, large; 2 Spratt curettes: straight, short; angled, long; 2 Weitlaner retractors, medium.

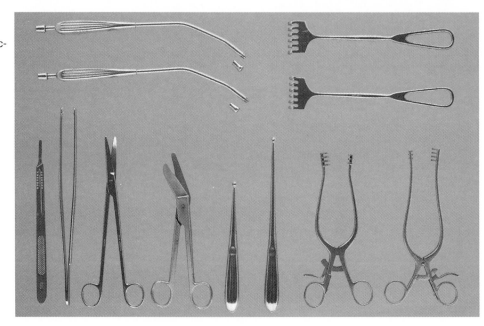

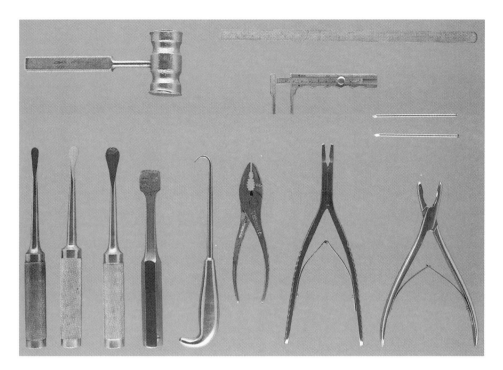

92-3 *Left, top,* 1 metal mallet. *Right, top to bottom,* 1 metal ruler, 12 inch; 1 inside/outside caliper; 2 Steinman pins, ⁹/₆₄. *Bottom, left to right,* 3 Cobb spinal elevators, small, medium, large; 1 Key periosteal elevator, 1 inch; 1 bone hook; 1 pliers; 1 Smith-Peterson laminectomy rongeur; 1 Luer bone rongeur.

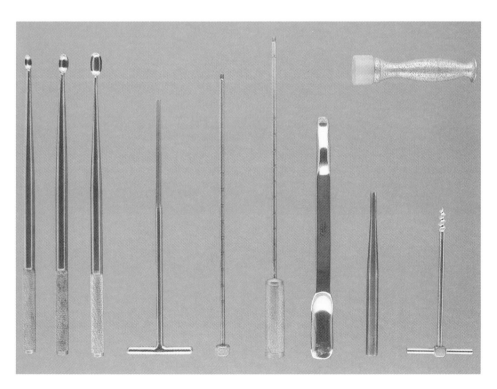

92-4 *Top right,* 1 prosthesis driver. *Bottom, left to right,* 3 Richards bone curettes, long, assorted sizes; 1 tapered T-handle femoral shaft reamer; 1 Buck's cement restrictor inserter; 1 Stryker cement restrictor inserter; 1 Murphy bone lever or skid; 1 impactor; 1 corkscrew femoral head remover.

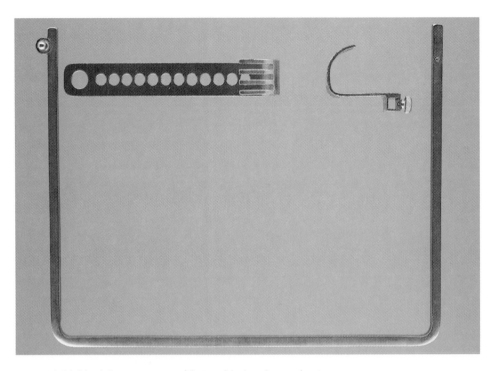

92-5 Initial incision retractor with two blades, long, short.

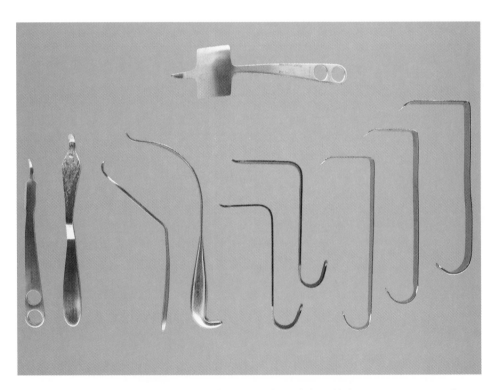

92-6 *Top,* 1 Holman retractor, large. *Bottom, left to right,* 1 Holman retractor, small; 3 Cobra retractors: straight, front view; angled and slightly angled, side view; side views 2 Taylor spinal retractors, black finish: short, long; 3 Hibbs laminectomy retractors, small, medium, large.

93

Hip Retractors and Instruments

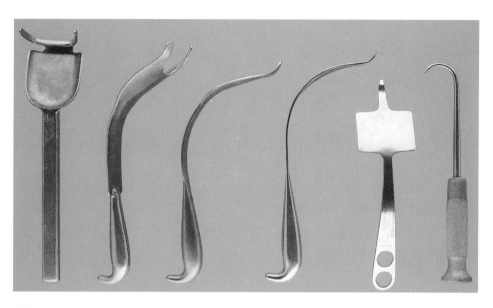

93-1 *Left to right,* 1 Antler retractor, front view; 1 double Cobra retractor, side view; 2 blunt Cobra retractors, side view; 1 Holman retractor, front view; 1 bone hook.

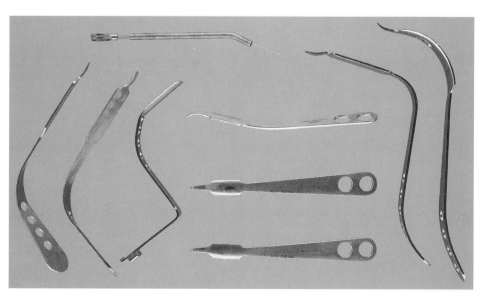

93-2 *Top,* 1 flexible depth gauge. *Bottom, left to right,* 2 anterior retractors, left, right; 1 superior retractor; 3 Holman retractors, narrow, side view, front view; 1 posterior/inferior retractor; 1 femoral retractor.

ADD BASIC TOTAL HIP SET AND HIP RETRACTORS

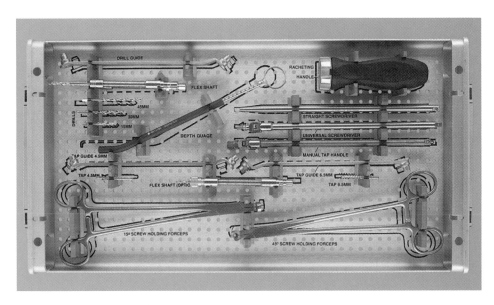

94-1 Instruments (Trilogy acetabular).

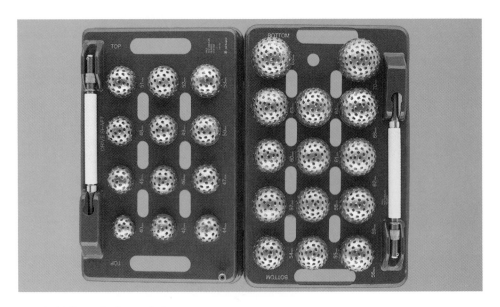

94-2 Hall surgical acetabular reamer set.

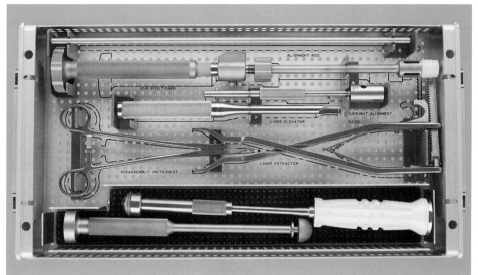

94-3 Shell provisionals and acetabular instruments.

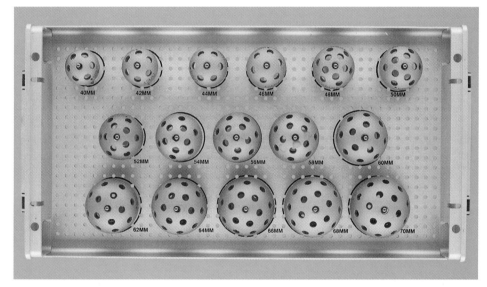

94-4 Shell provisionals and acetabulars.

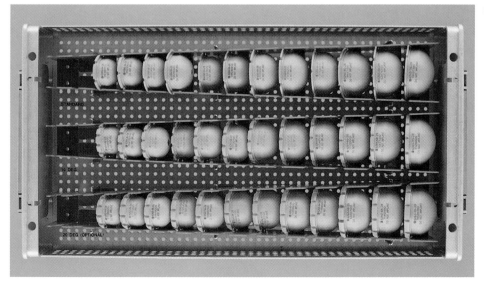

94-5 Linear provisionals.

94-6 General instruments—stem.

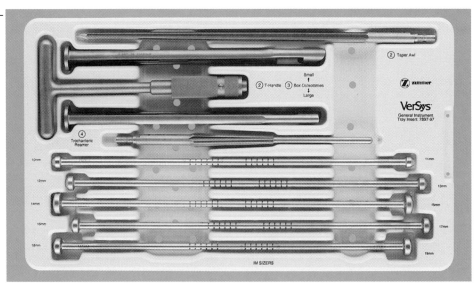

94-7 General instruments—femoral.

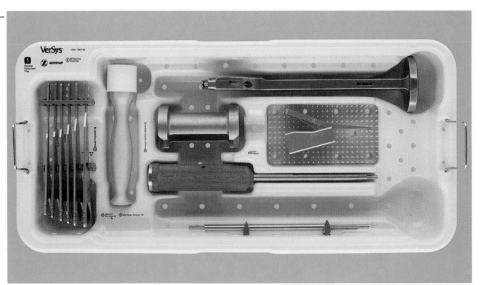

94-8 Rasp tray.

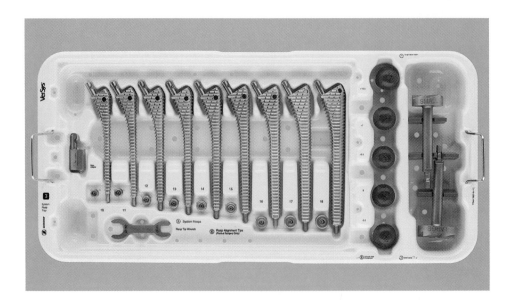

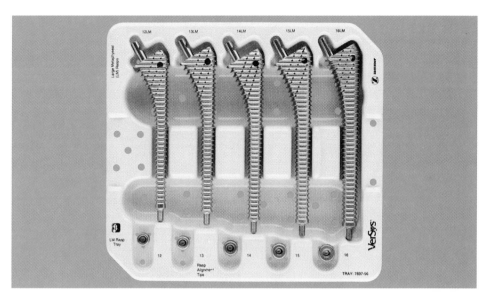

94-9 Large metaphyseal tray.

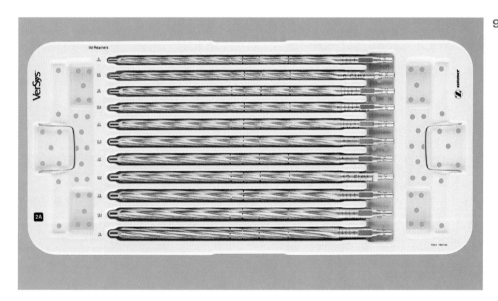

94-10 Reamer tray 2 A.

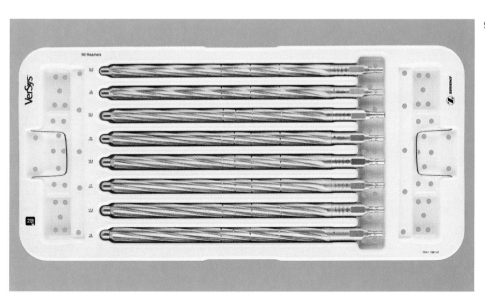

94-11 Reamer tray 2 B.

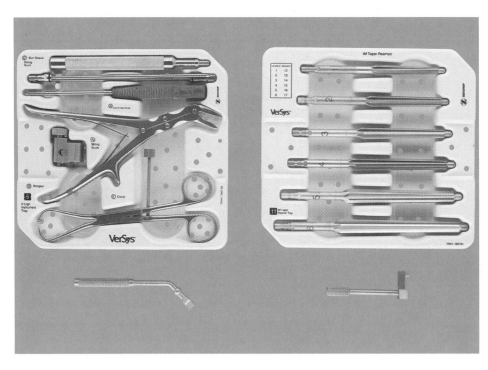

94-12 *Left to right,* V-Lign instrument tray; intramedullary (IM) taper reamers.

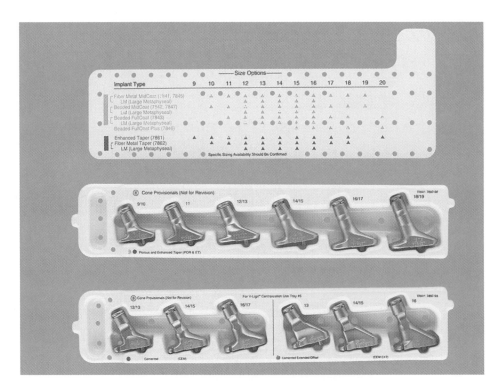

94-13 Cone provisionals: size options: *top,* porous and enhanced taper; *bottom, left,* cemented; *bottom, right,* cemented extended offset.

Total Hip Prosthesis (VerSys Hip System)

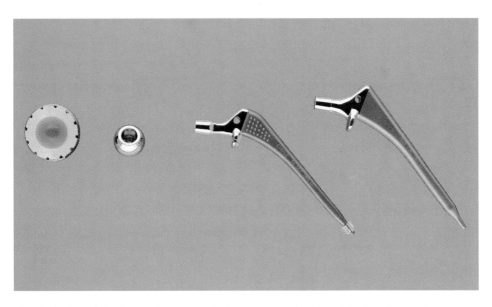

95-1 *Left to right,* 1 acetabular prothesis; 1 femoral head prothesis; 2 femoral stem protheses: plain, cemented.

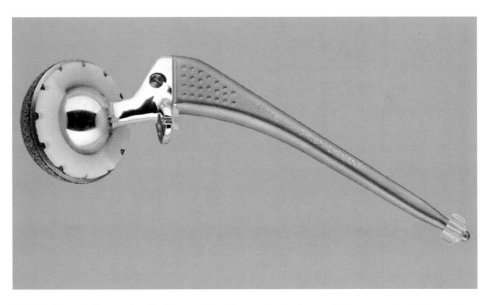

95-2 Acetabular prothesis; femoral head prosthesis; femoral stem prosthesis together.

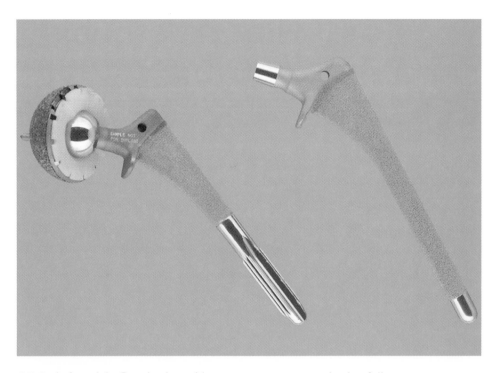

95-3 *Left to right,* Prosthesis—midcoat porous stem; prosthesis—fully porous stem.

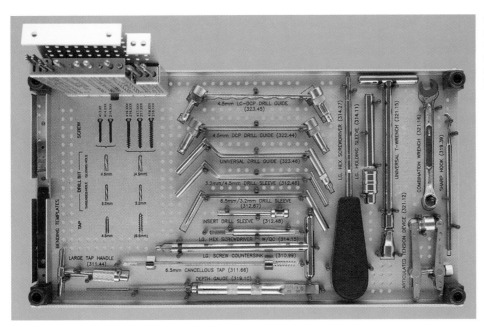

96-1 Association for the Study of Internal Fixation (ASIF) basic low contact–dynamic compression plate (LC-DCP) and DCP instrument set.

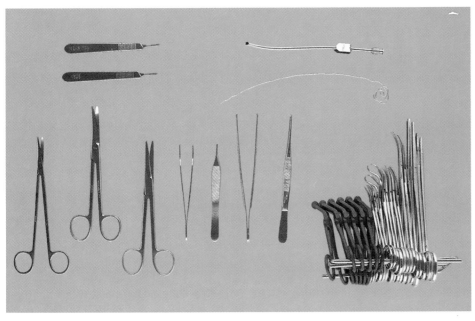

96-2 *Top, left to right,* 2 Bard Parker knife handles, No. 3; 1 Adson suction tube, stylet, 14 Fr. *Bottom, left to right,* 1 Metzenbaum scissors, 7 inch; 2 Mayo dissecting scissors, curved, straight; 2 Adson tissue forceps with teeth (1 × 2), front view, side view; 2 thumb tissue forceps with teeth (1 × 2), front view, side view; 6 paper drape clips; 2 Halstead mosquito hemostatic forceps; 2 Backhaus towel forceps; 4 Crile hemostatic forceps, 5½ inch; 2 tonsil hemostatic forceps; 2 Ochsner hemostatic forceps; 2 Crile Wood needle holders, 7 inch.

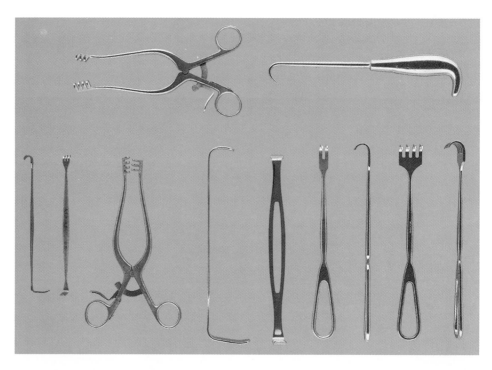

96-3 *Top, left to right,* 1 Weitlaner retractor, sharp, medium; 1 bone hook. *Bottom, left to right,* 2 Miller-Senn retractors, side view, front view; 1 Weitlaner retractor, sharp, medium; 2 Army Navy retractors, side view, front view; 4 Volkmann retractors: 2 2 pronged, sharp; 2 4 pronged, sharp; side view, front view.

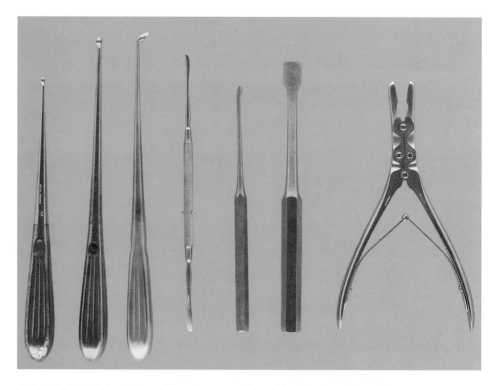

96-4 *Left to right,* 3 Spratt (Brun) curettes, long: No. 00, 2, and 3 angled; Freer double-ended elevator; 2 Key periosteal elevators: $1/4$ inch side view, $1/2$ inch front view; 1 Ruskin ronguer.

ASIF Mini–Fragment Instruments

ADD TO ASIF BASIC SET

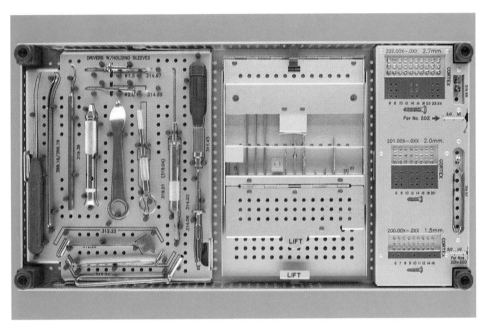

97-1 ASIF mini–fragment set (labeled).

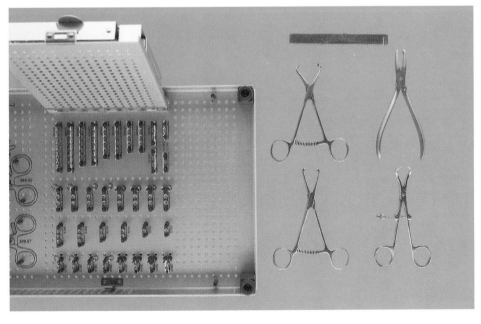

97-2 *Left to right, bottom of tray under drills.* Some instrumentation from tray.

ASIF Small Fragment Instruments

ADD TO ASIF BASIC SET

98-1 ASIF small fragment set (labeled).

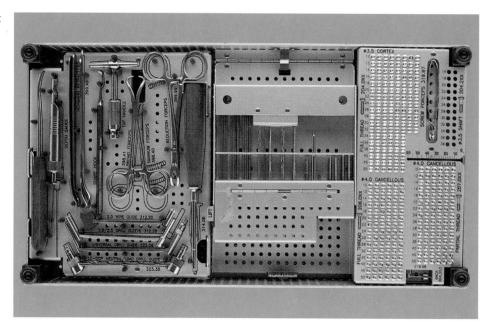

98-2 *Left to right, bottom of tray under drills.* Some instrumentation from tray.

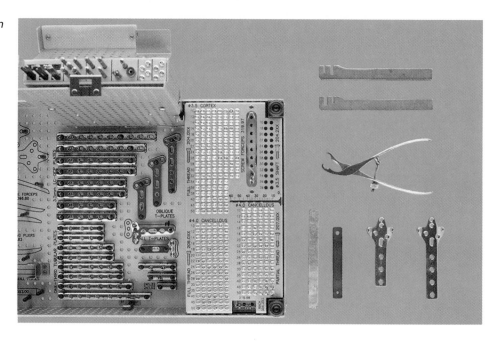

ASIF Basic LC-DCP and DCP Instrument Set

ADD TO ASIF BASIC SET

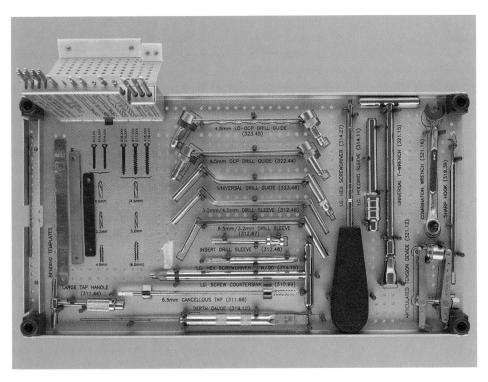

99-1 ASIF basic LC-DCP and DCP instruments.

ASIF Standard Screws

ADD ASIF BASIC SET AND ASIF INSTRUMENTS

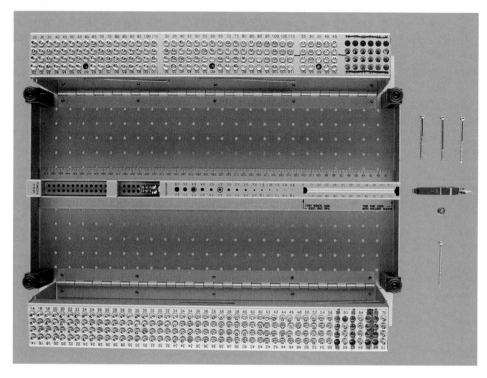

100-1 ASIF standard screw set in tray (labeled) and some screws from tray to right.

ASIF Standard Plates

ADD ASIF BASIC SET, ASIF STANDARD INSTRUMENTS, AND ASIF STANDARD SCREWS

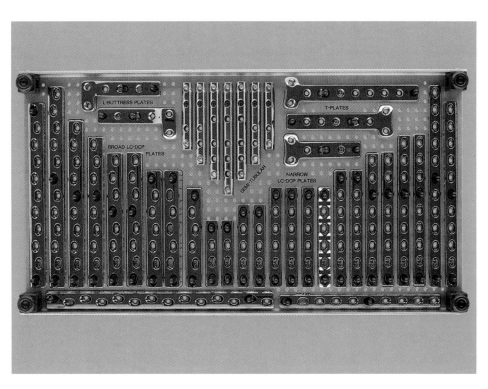

101-1 ASIF standard plate set in tray (labeled).

Dynamic Hip Screw (DHS) Instruments and Screws

ADD TO OPEN REDUCTION SET

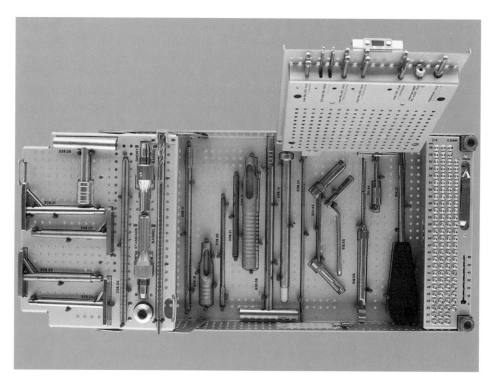

102-1 DHS instrument and screw set (labeled).

ADD OPEN REDUCTION SET, DHS INSTRUMENTS, AND SCREWS

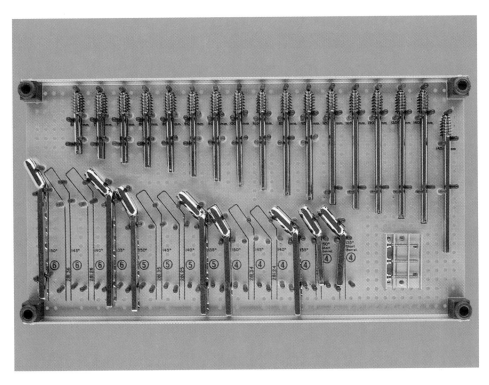

103-1 DHS implants in tray (labeled).

TSRH Spinal Rodding Set

ADD OPEN REDUCTION SET

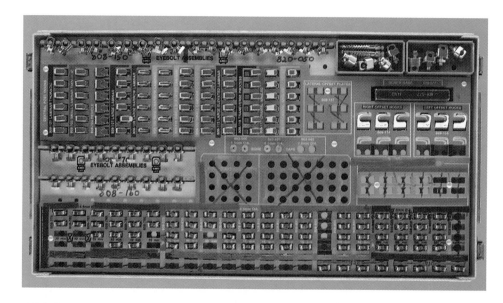

104-1 Texas Scottish Rite Hospital (TSRH) implant tray (labeled).

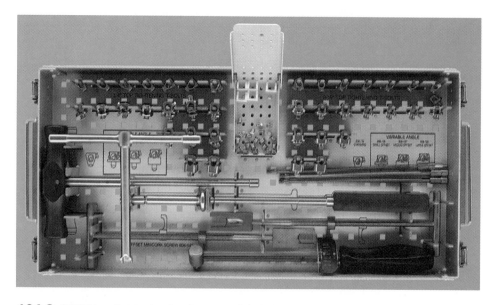

104-2 TSRH top tightening implant tray (labeled).

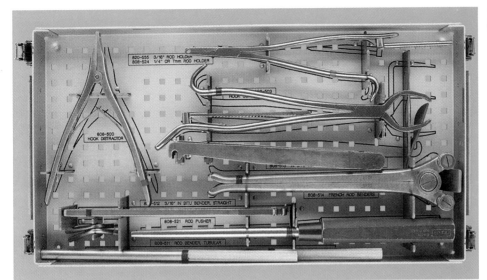

104-3 TSRH bending tray (labeled).

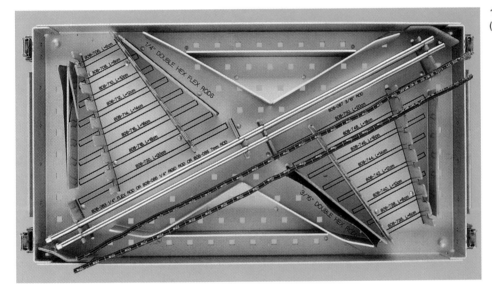

104-4 TSRH rod tray (labeled).

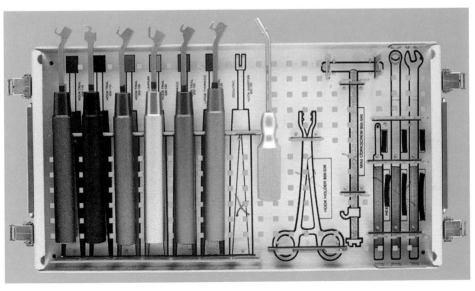

104-5 TSRH pediatric instrument bottom tray (labeled).

104-6 TSRH pediatric instrument top tray (labeled).

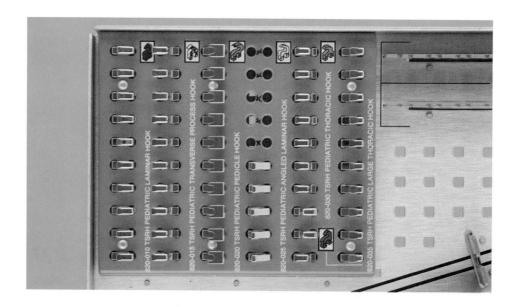

104-7 TSRH hook trials (labeled).

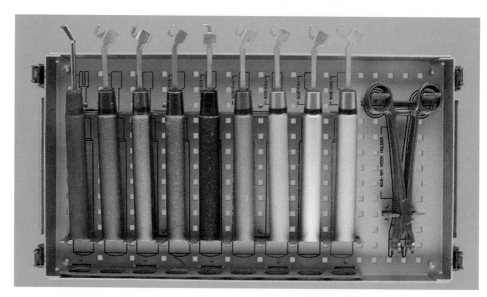

104-8 TSRH cross link tray (labeled).

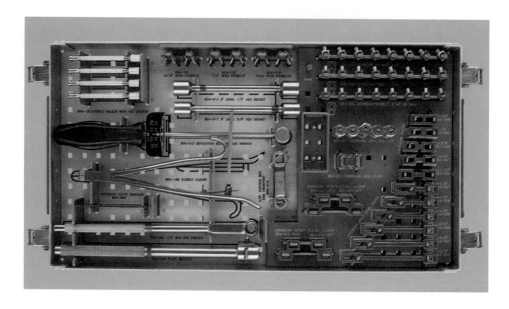

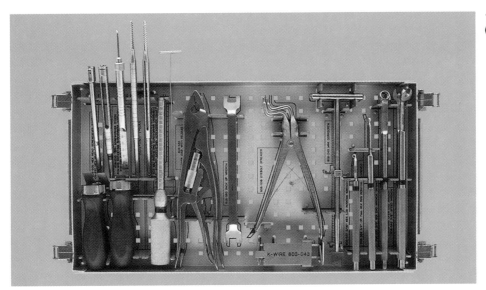

104-9 TSRH wrench tray (labeled).

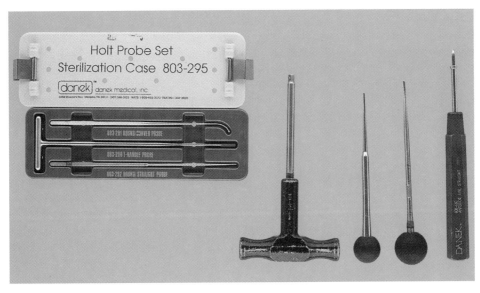

104-10 *Left, top to bottom,* Holt probe set: curved probe, T-handle probe, round/straight probe. *Bottom, left to right,* 1 T-handle wrench; 2 probes (Acromed); 1 anterior awl, straight.

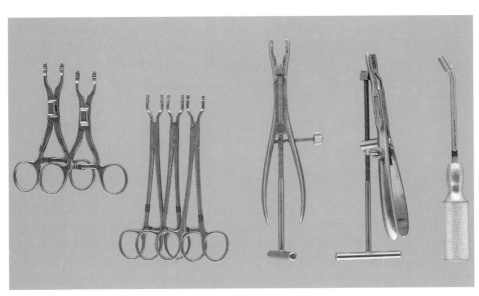

104-11 *Left to right,* 2 mini–hook holders with attachments; 3 hook holders, four pegged; 2 hook holders with rod movers; 1 hook inserter.

104-12 *Left to right,*
1 Harrington outrigger (3
pieces); 1 Harrington outrigger nut, pin, wrench; 1 large
compressor; 1 curved
spreader (Sofamor); 1 large
distractor.

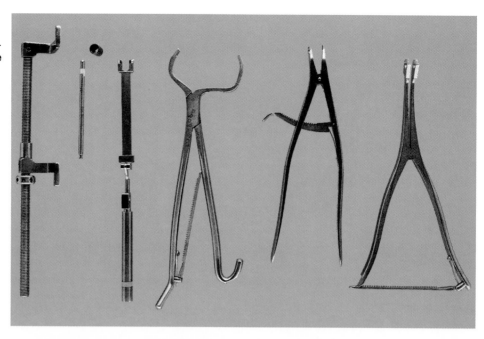

104-13 Rod cutter.

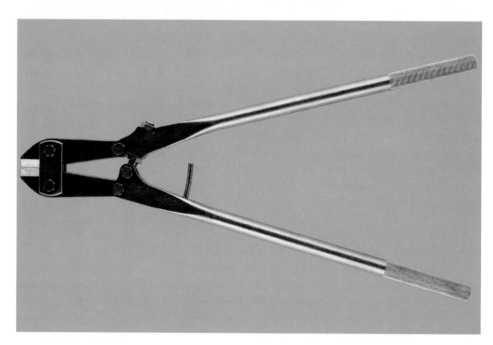

Amputation-of-an-Extremity Instruments

ADD SOFT TISSUE SET

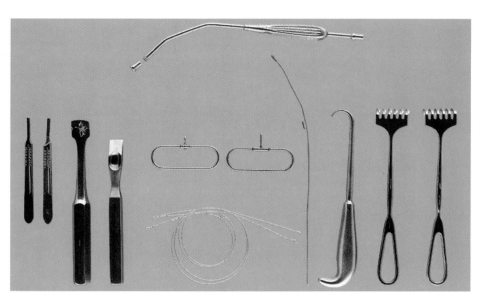

105-1 *Top,* 1 Yankauer suction tube and tip. *Left to right,* 2 Bard Parker knife handles, No. 4; 1 Key periosteal elevator, large; Gigli saw: 3 blades, 2 handles, 1 guide; 1 bone hook; 2 Volkmann retractors, 6 pronged, sharp.

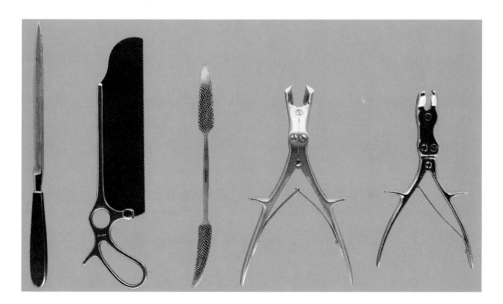

105-2 *Left to right,* 1 Liston amputation knife; 1 Saterlee amputation saw; 1 Putti bone rasp, double-ended; 1 Stille-Horsley bone cutting forceps, double-action; 1 Stille-Luer rongeur.

ASIF Mini–Fixation Set

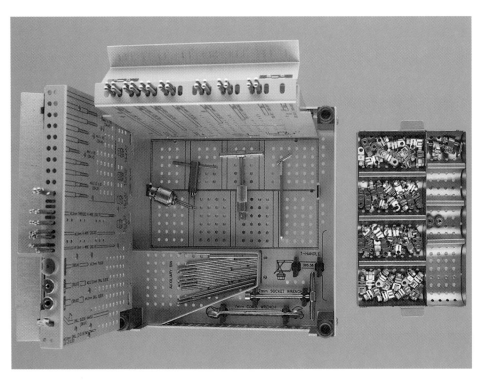

106-1 ASIF external fixator miniset.

ASIF Pelvic Instrument Set

ADD SOFT TISSUE SET

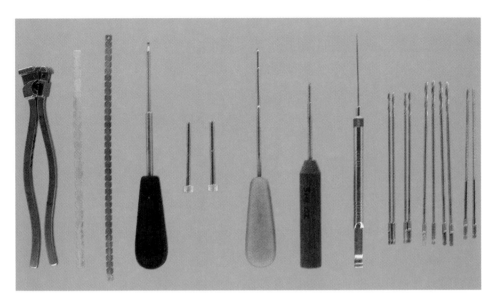

107-1 *Left to right,* 1 plate bender; 2 pelvic plate-bending templates, long; 1 small hexagonal screwdriver; 2 drill guides, long, 2.5, 3.5 mm; 1 small hexagonal screwdriver, long, large handled; 1 small hexagonal screwdriver, regular; 1 depth gauge; 2 drill bits, 2.5 × 180 mm; 4 drill bits, 3.5 × 170 mm; 2 taps, 3.5 × 180 mm.

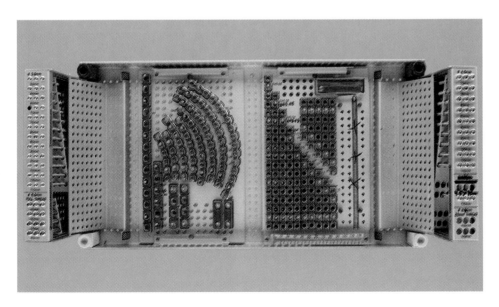

107-2 ASIF pelvic implant set.

ASIF Condylar Instruments

ADD SOFT TISSUE SET

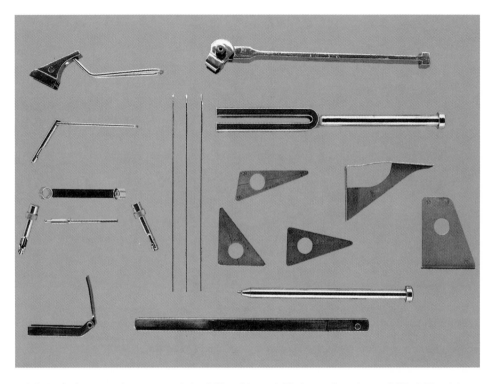

108-1 *Left, top to bottom,* 1 triple drill guide; 1 drill sleeve for plates; DCP drill guide (four pieces); 1 chisel guide, 16 mm. *Middle,* 3 guide pins. *Right, top to bottom,* 1 inserter/extractor; 1 slotted hammer; 3 triangular positioning plates, assorted sizes; 1 condylar plate guide; 1 quadrangular positioning plate; 1 impactor; 1 seating chisel.

ASIF Angular Blade Plate Set

ADD SOFT TISSUE SET

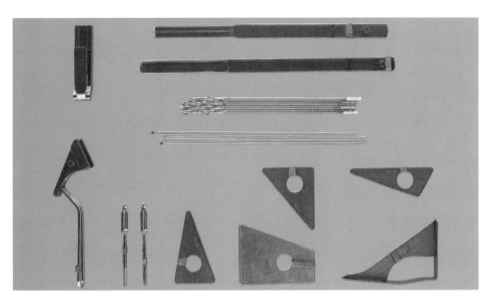

109-1 *Left, top to bottom,* 1 chisel guide/adjuster, angular; 1 triple drill guide. *Right, top to bottom,* 1 seating chisel–adolescent; 1 seating chisel; 4 quick-coupling drill bits, 4.5 mm; 4 guide pins. *Bottom, left to right,* 2 routers; 3 triangular positioning plates, assorted sizes; 1 quadrangular positioning plate; 1 condylar plate guide.

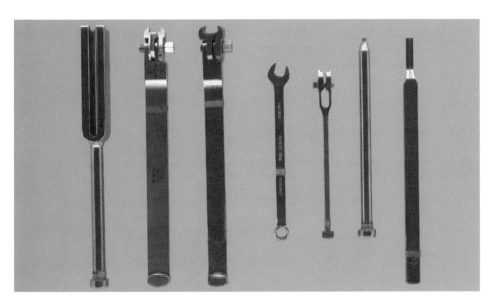

109-2 *Left to right,* 1 slotted hammer; 1 impact adolescent plate; 1 inserter/extractor; 1 wrench, 11 mm; 1 insert-bifurcated plate; 1 impactor; 1 seating chisel–infant.

ASIF Cannulated Screw Set

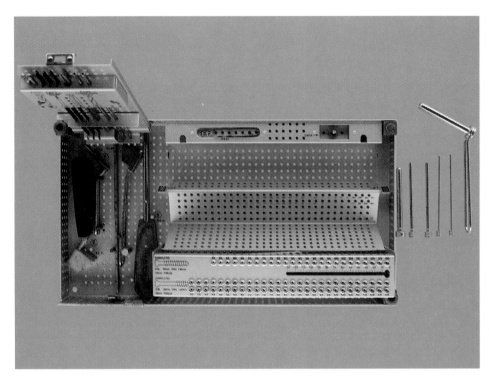

110-1 Synthes cannulated screw set (labeled).

ASIF Medullary Instruments

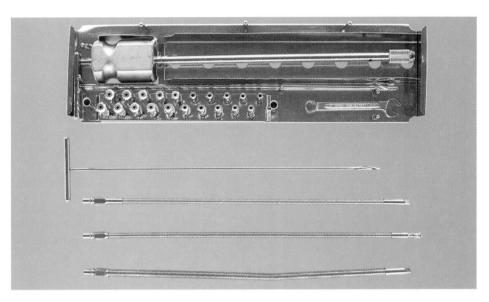

111-1 *Top,* Tray that includes reamer heads, flexible shafts and reamer, ram, cannulated guide rod. *Middle,* wrench. *Bottom,* 3 hand reamers.

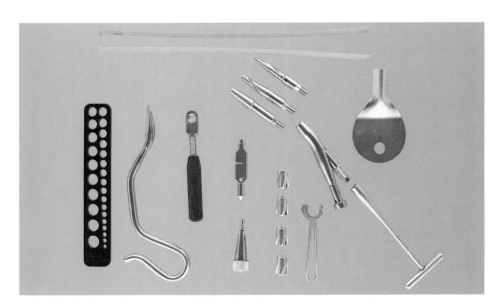

111-2 *Top,* 2 plastic medullary tubes. *Bottom, left to right,* 1 diameter gauge; 1 awl; 1 socket wrench for conical bolts. *Middle, top to bottom,* 3 threaded conical bolts; 1 guide handle for nails; 1 quick-coupling adapter; 4 reamer heads, assorted sizes; 1 holder for reaming rod and guide shaft; 1 curved driver (2 pieces); 1 tissue protector.

ASIF Universal Distractor Set

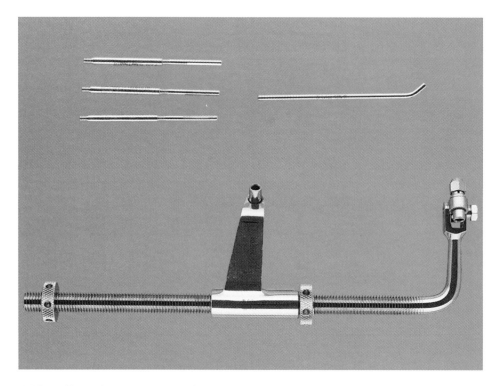

112-1 *Top to bottom,* 3 connecting bolts; 1 pin wrench; 1 distractor.

Titanium-Unreamed Femoral Nail Instruments

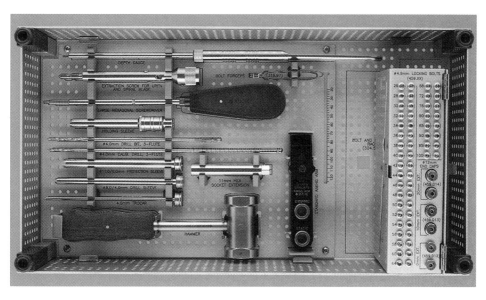

113-1 Ti-unreamed femoral nail instrument set: bottom tray (labeled).

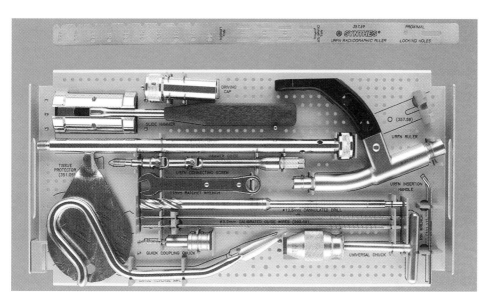

113-2 Ti-unreamed femoral nail instrument set: top tray (labeled).

114

Synthes Unreamed Tibial Nails

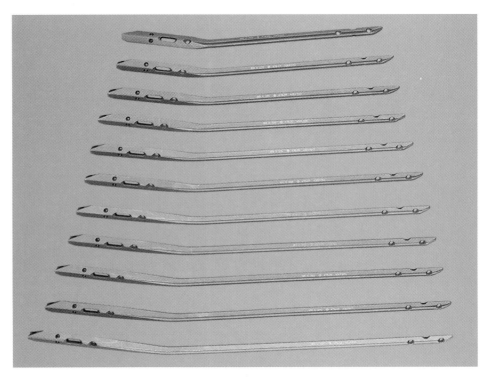

114-1 Synthes unreamed tibial nail set, assorted sizes.

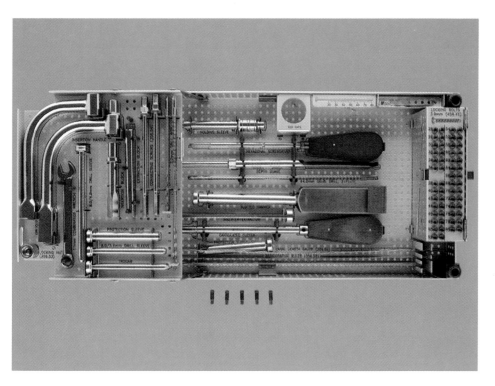

115

Synthes Unreamed Tibial Nail Insertion and Locking Instruments

115-1 Synthes unreamed tibial nail insertion and locking set (labeled).

Unit Ten

GENITOURINARY PROCEDURES

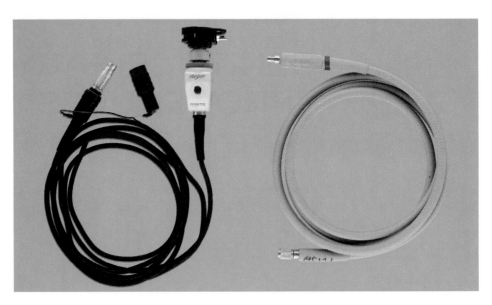

116-1 Standard cystoscopy set: camera, light cable.

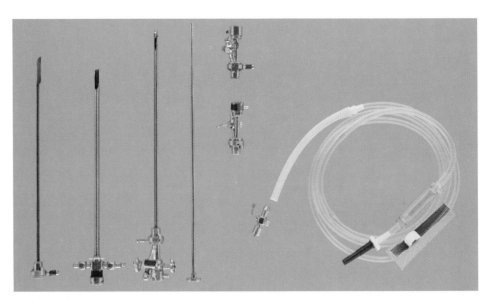

116-2 *Left to right,* 1 obturator; 1 cystoscope sheath; 1 catheter deflecting mechanism with two instrument channels; 1 obturator for cystoscope. *Top to bottom,* 2 Storz short telescope bridges; 1 cystoscope stopcock at end of fluid cord.

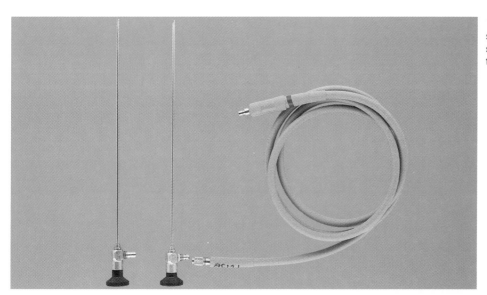

116-3 *Left to right,* 1 telescope, 30 degree; 1 telescope, 70 degree; 1 fiberoptic light cable.

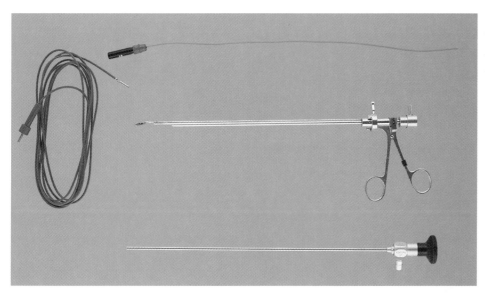

116-4 *Left,* 1 cautery cord. *Top to bottom,* 1 Bugbee electrode; 1 biopsy forceps; 1 telescope, 0 degree.

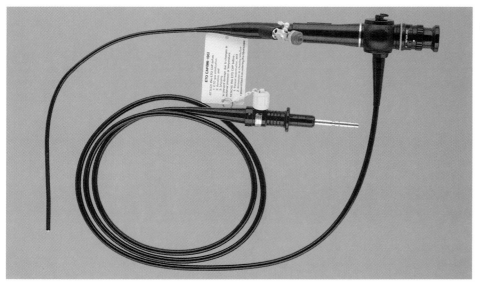

116-5 Olympus flexible cystoscope with cord.

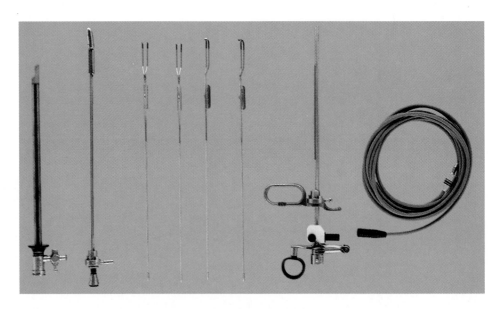

117-1 *Left to right,* 1 resecting sheath, 27 Fr; 1 deflecting obturator; 2 resecting loops; 1 rollar ball electrode; 1 coagulating electrode with pointed end; 1 resectoscope working element; 1 high-frequency cautery.

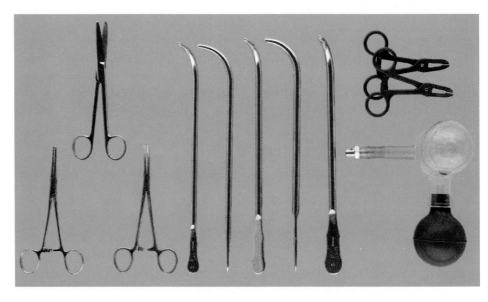

117-2 *Left to right, top to bottom,* 1 Mayo dissecting scissors, curved; 2 Crile hemostatic forceps, straight, curved; 5 Van Buren urethral sounds, male, sizes 8 to 16; 2 paper drape clips; 1 Ellik evacutor.

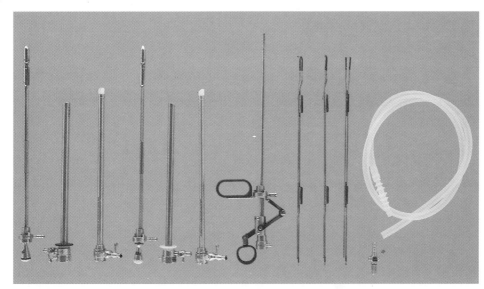

117-3 *Left to right,* Low-pressure resecting set: 1 deflecting obturator; 1 resecting sheath, 28 Fr; 1 resecting sheath, 28 Fr, insulated; 1 deflecting obturator; 1 resecting sheath, 26 Fr; 1 resecting sheath, 26 Fr, insulated; 1 working element; 3 electrodes, sharp, ball, loop; 1 stopcock and tubing.

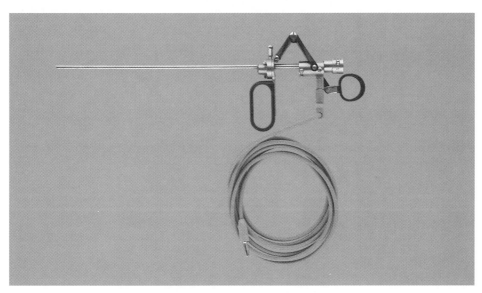

117-4 Working element and connecting cord.

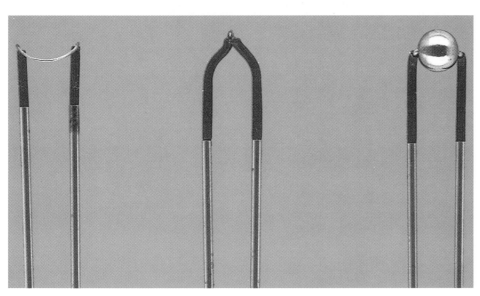

117-5 *Left to right,* enlarged tips: 1 cutting electrode with round wire; 1 cutting electrode with pointed end; 1 coagulating electrode with ball end.

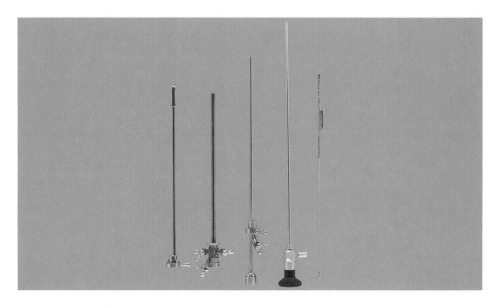

118-1 *Left to right,* 1 obturator; 1 urethroscope sheath; 1 telescope adapting bridge; 1 telescope, 0 degree; 1 urethrotome blade.

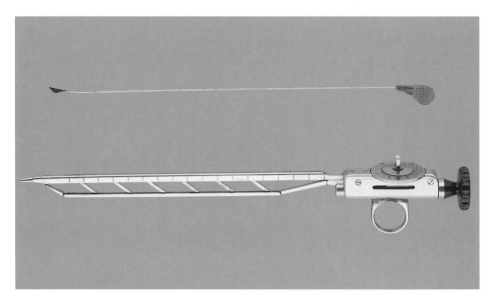

118-2 *Top to bottom,* Otis urethrotome: blade, urethrotome.

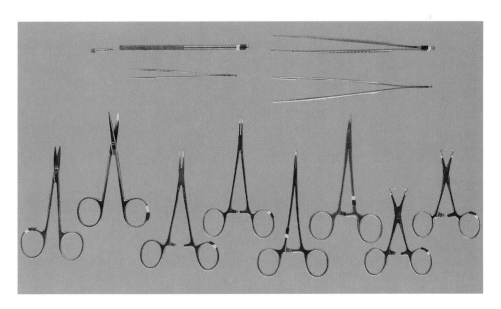

119-1 *Top to bottom, left to right,* 1 Beaver knife handle, knurled, with tip; 1 jeweler's forceps; 2 DeBakey Autraugrip tissue forceps, short. *Bottom, left to right,* 1 iris scissors, straight, sharp; 1 Stevens tenotomy scissors; 4 Providence hemostatic forceps; 2 Backhaus towel forceps.

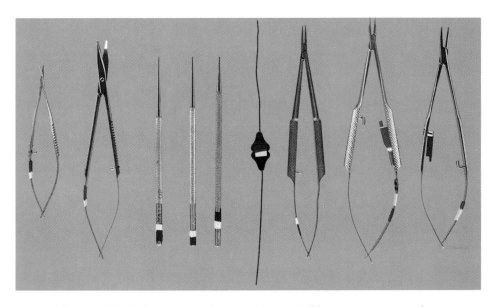

119-2 *Left to right,* 1 Vannas capsulotomy scissors; 1 Westcott tenotomy scissors; 3 Henle probes, assorted sizes; 1 lacrimal probes, 0-00; 1 titanium micro–needle holder, nonlocking; 1 Barraquer needle holder, extra delicate, tapered, curved, with lock; 1 Troutman tier needle holder with lock.

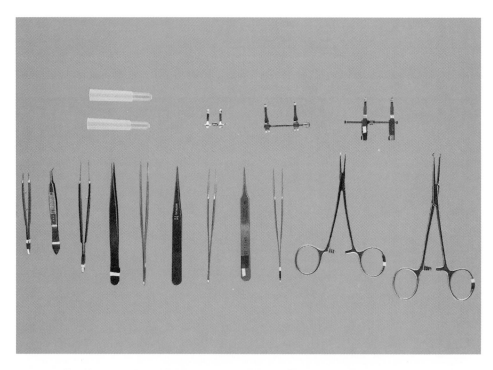

119-3 *Top, left to right,* 2 chamber maintainers; 1 Silher vasovasotomy clamp; 2 Strauch vasovasotomy approximators, hinged, small, large; 2 McPherson tying forceps, angled, front view, side view; 1 Castroviejo suturing forceps, 0.12 mm, front view; 3 jeweler's forceps, No. 3, side view, front view, side view; 2 jeweler's forceps, No. 4, front view, side view; 1 jeweler's forceps, No. 5, front view; 1 Snowden-Pencer dissecting forceps; 1 Snowden-Pencer fixation forceps.

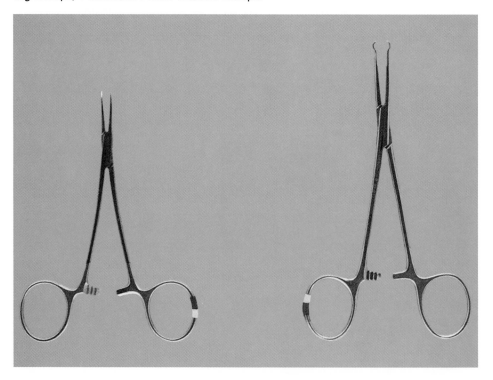

119-4 *Left to right,* 1 Snowden-Pencer dissecting forceps; 1 Snowden-Pencer fixation forceps.

Unit Eleven

ORAL, MAXILLARY, AND FACIAL SURGERY

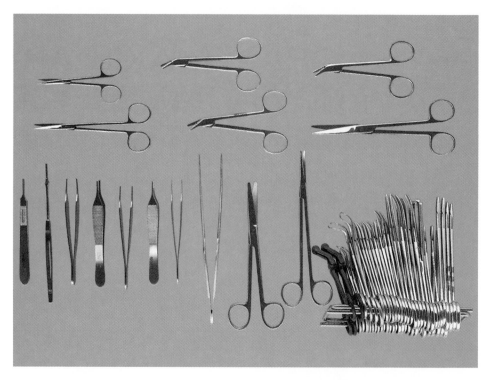

120-1 *Top, left to right,* 1 Stevens tenotomy scissors, curved; 1 plastic scissors, straight, sharp; 3 wire(-cutting) scissors; 1 Mayo dissecting scissors, straight. *Bottom, left to right,* 2 Bard Parker knife handles, No. 3, No. 7; 2 Adson tissue forceps with teeth (1 × 2), front view, side view; 2 Adson tissue forceps without teeth, front view, side view; 1 Brown-Adson tissue forceps with teeth (7 × 7), front view; 1 bayonet dressing forceps, 7½ inch; 1 Mayo dissecting scissors, curved; 1 Metzenbaum scissors; 2 paper drape clips; 2 Backhaus towel forceps, small; 2 Backhaus towel forceps; 6 Halstead mosquito hemostatic forceps, curved; 2 Halstead mosquito hemostatic forceps, straight; 2 Providence hemostatic forceps, curved; 2 Halstead hemostatic forceps, straight; 4 Crile hemostatic forceps, curved; 2 Allis tissue forceps; 2 Webster needle holders, 4 inch; 2 Crile Wood needle holders, 6 inch; 2 Johnson needle holders, 6 inch.

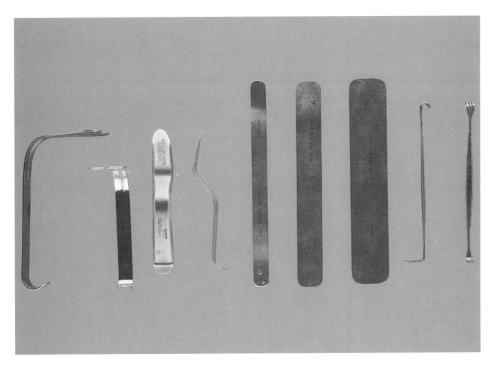

120-2 *Left to right,* 2 Wieder tongue retractors: large, small, side view, front view; 2 University of Minnesota cheek retractors, front view, side view; 3 ribbon retractors, assorted sizes; 2 Senn-Kanavel retractors, side view, front view.

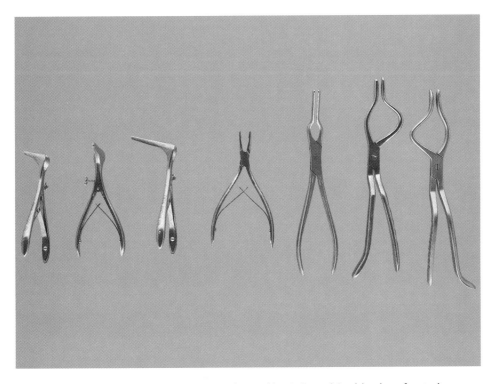

120-3 *Left to right,* 3 Cottle nasal speculums: No. 1, 2, and 3; side view, front view, side view; 1 Friedman rongeur, single action; 1 Asche forceps; 2 Rowe disimpaction forceps, left, right.

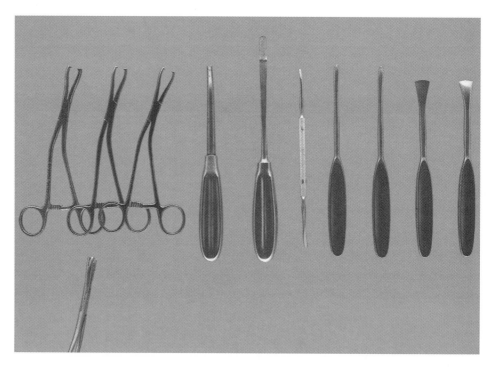

120-4 *Left to right,* 4 Dingman bone-holding forceps, tip of 4th at bottom; 1 Dingman zygoma elevator; 1 Gilles malar elevator; 1 Freer elevator; 2 Langenbeck elevators; 2 Langenbeck periosteal elevators, straight, angled.

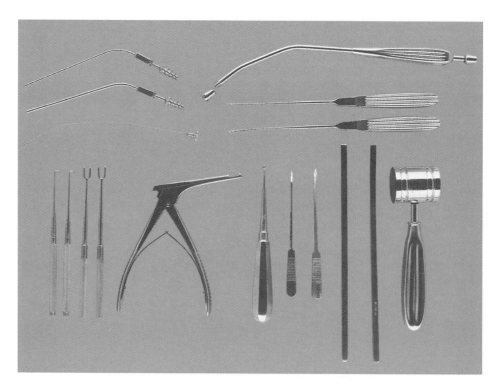

120-5 *Top, left to right,* 2 Frazier suction tubes with stylet; 1 Yankauer suction tube with tip; 2 zygomatic arch awls. *Bottom, left to right,* 2 Joseph skin hooks, single; 2 Joseph skin hooks, double; 1 Kerrison rongeur, 90-degree upbite; 1 Lucas curette, No. 0, short; 2 mandibular awls; 2 Cottle osteotomes, curved, straight; 1 metal mallet.

121

Orthognathic Instruments

ADD FACIAL FRACTURE SET

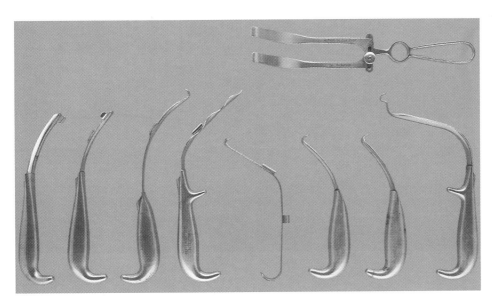

121-1 *Top,* 1 Burton retractor, double. *Left to right,* 2 Bauer retractors, left, right; 1 Joseph Coronoid self-retaining retractor; 1 Petri pterygoid retractor; 1 channel retractor; 2 general purpose retractors; 1 Kent Wood adjustable retractor.

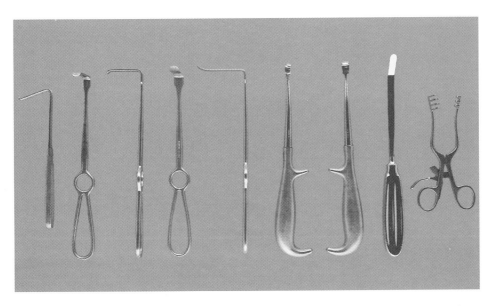

121-2 *Left to right,* 1 piriform rim retractor; 2 Langenbeck retractors, front view, side view; 2 Langenbeck retractors, up-curved tip, front view, side view; 2 pterygo masseteric sling strippers, small, medium; 1 Gilles malar elevator; 1 Weitlaner retractor, 5 inch, blunt pronged.

121-3 *Left to right,*
2 roller compressions with
metal trocar points above,
small, large; 1 trocar cannula (with trocar); 1 trocar
with handle; 1 holding forceps; 2 dental mirrors, No.
5; 2 cheek retractors;
1 mandibular reduction
forceps.

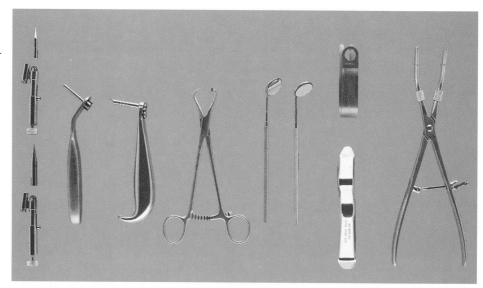

121-4 *Left to right,* 1 drill
guide; 1 nasal ball end
osteotome; 5 osteotomes:
3 straight, 4, 6, and 8mm;
angled, 6 mm; curved,   8
mm; 1 Parkes osteotome; 1
sagittal splitting osteotome;
1 Crile Wood needle holder,
curved, 6 inch; 1 Coronoid
match retractor.

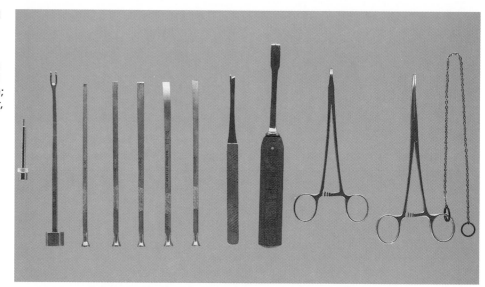

121-5 *Top,* 2 trocar cannulas. *Bottom, left to right,*
1 caliper; 1 condylar stripper; 1 Byrd screw; 2 zygomatic arch awls; 1 Freer elevator double-ended; 1
periosteal elevator; 1 chisel.

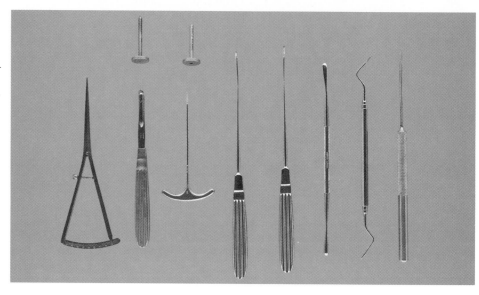

Titanium 2.0 mm
Micro–Fixation System

ADD FACIAL FRACTURE SET. ORTHOGNATHIC INSTRUMENTS MAY BE NEEDED

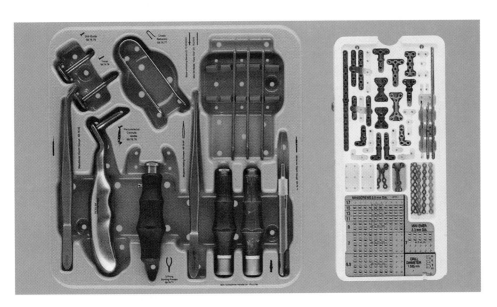

122-1 Titanium 2.0 mm micro–fixation system instrumentation, 2 of 3 trays (labeled).

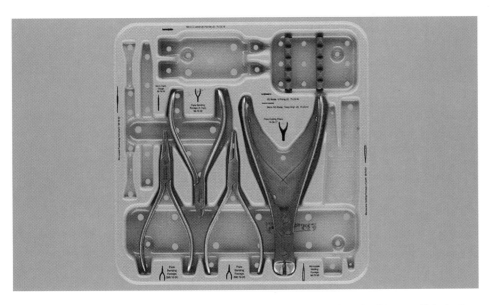

122-2 Titanium 2.0 mm micro–fixation system instrumentation, 3 of 3 trays (labeled).

Tooth Impaction Set

123-1 *Top to bottom, left to right,* 1 Locklin scissors; 1 Metzenbaum scissors, 5 inch; 1 Mayo dissecting scissors, straight; 1 Astra aspirating syringe. *Bottom, left to right,* 1 Bard Parker knife handle, No. 3; 2 Adson tissue forceps: with teeth (1 × 2); without teeth; 2 Russian tissue forceps, short, front view, side view; 1 bayonet dressing forceps; 2 Halstead mosquito hemostatic forceps, curved; 2 Crile hemostatic forceps, 6½ inch; 1 Crile Wood needle holder, 7 inch.

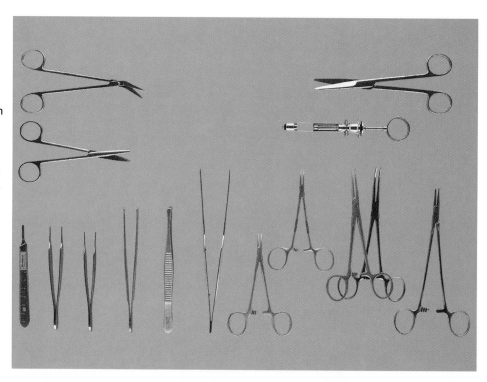

123-2 *Top,* 1 Yankauer suction tube with tip. *Bottom, left to right,* 1 double-ended retractor; 1 Freer elevator double-ended; 1 Lucas curette, short, straight, No. 0; 1 ball-ended nasal osteotome; 1 Gardner mallet; 2 Frazier suction tubes, No. 6, with stylet; 2 Frazier suction tubes, angled, with stylet.

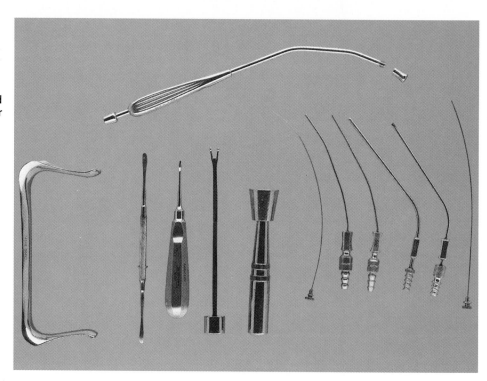

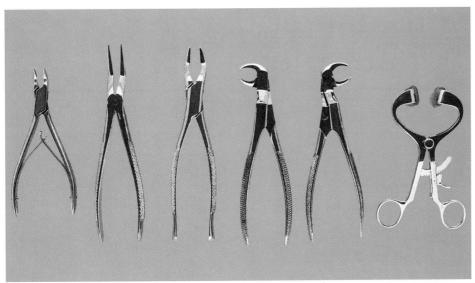

123-3 *Left to right,* 1 single-action rongeur, small; 1 root and splinter forceps; 1 upper incisor and cuspid forceps; 2 Roturier lower third molar forceps, left, right; 1 Molt mouth gag.

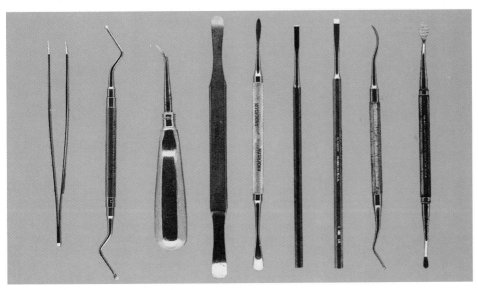

123-4 *Left to right,* 1 cotton plier; 1 Crane pick elevator; 1 Lucas curette, No. 10; 1 Seldin periosteal elevator; 1 Freer elevator double-ended; 2 carbide chisels: bi-beveled, single beveled; 2 bone files (rasps), side view, front view.

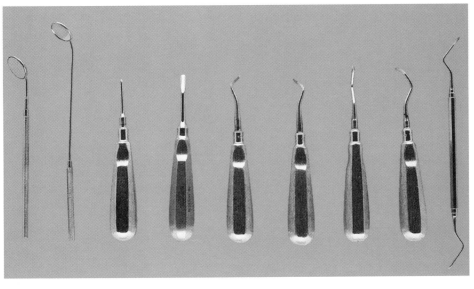

123-5 *Left to right,* 2 laryngeal mirrors, No. 5, No. 4; 4 elevators: No. 1, 34, 190, and 191; 2 Miller elevators: No. 71, No. 72; 1 Davis root teaser, No. 11.

124

Temporomandibular Joint (TMJ) Instruments

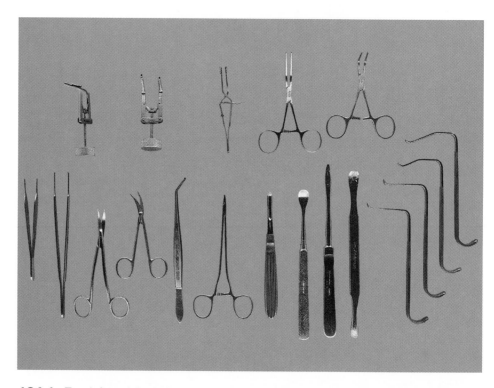

124-1 *Top, left to right,* 2 Wilks self-retaining retractors, left, right; 1 Walton self-retaining retractor; 2 angled vascular clamps: 45 degrees, 90 degrees. *Bottom, left to right,* 1 Adson tissue forceps with teeth (1 × 2); 1 Gerald tissue forceps with teeth (1 × 2); 1 pharyngeal scissors, curved; 1 sickle scissors; 1 Cushing tissue forceps with lock, angled; 1 Sarot needle holder; 1 condylar stripper; 1 Hu-Friedy elevator, No. 2; 1 periosteal elevator, No. 9; 1 periosteal elevator, double-ended; 4 condylar retractors: 2 superior, posterior, anterior; assorted sizes.

Unit Twelve

PLASTIC SURGERY

125

Minor Plastic Set

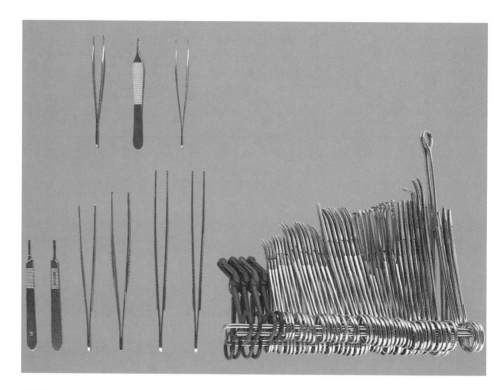

125-1 *Top, left to right,* 2 Adson tissue forceps with teeth (1 × 2), front view, side view; 1 Brown Adson tissue forceps with teeth (7 × 7), front view. *Bottom, left to right,* 2 Bard Parker knife handles, No. 3; 2 DeBakey Autraugrip tissue forceps, short; 2 Cushing tissue forceps with teeth (1 × 2); 4 paper drape clips; 6 Halstead mosquito hemostatic forceps, curved; 1 Halstead mosquito hemostatic forceps, straight; 8 Crile hemostatic forceps, curved, 5½ inch; 1 Halstead hemostatic forceps, straight; 6 Crile hemostatic forceps, curved, 6½ inch; 4 Allis tissue forceps; 4 Babcock tissue forceps; 4 Ochsner hemostatic forceps, straight; 1 Westphal hemostatic forceps; 2 tonsil hemostatic forceps; 1 Foerster sponge forceps; 1 Johnson needle holder, 6 inch; 2 Crile Wood needle holders, 6 inch.

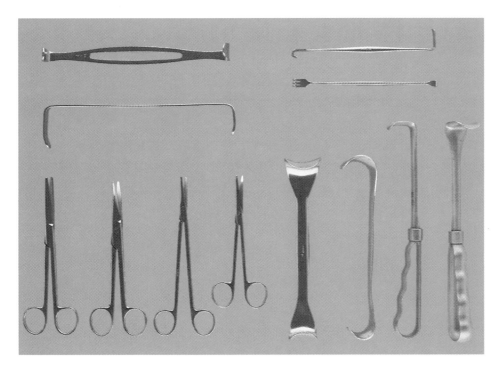

125-2 *Top, left to right,* 2 Army-Navy retractors, front view, side view; 2 Miller-Senn retractors, side view, front view. *Bottom, left to right,* 2 Mayo dissecting scissors, straight, curved; 2 Metzenbaum scissors, 7 inch, 5 inch; 2 Goelet retractors, front view, side view; 2 Richardson retractors, small, side view, front view.

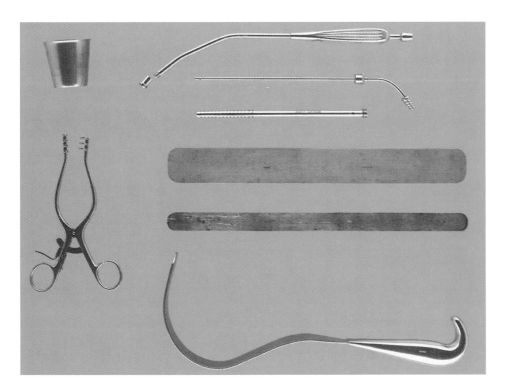

125-3 *Left, top to bottom,* 1 metal medicine cup, 2 oz.; 1 Weitlaner retractor, small. *Right, top to bottom,* 1 Yankauer suction tube with tip; 1 Poole abdominal suction tube with shield; 2 Ochsner malleable retractors, medium, narrow; 1 Deaver retractor, medium.

Skin Graft Instruments

ADD MINOR PLASTIC SET

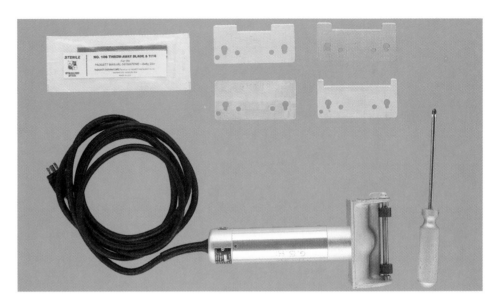

126-1 Padgett electric dermatome with disposable blade (left).

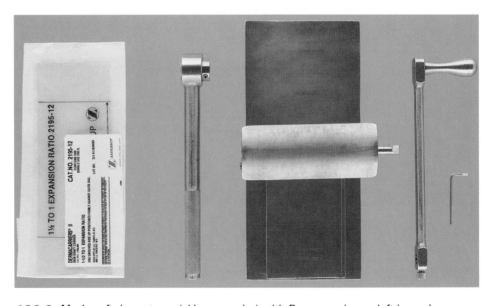

126-2 Meshgraft dermatome (skin expander) with Dermacarrier on left in package.

Unit Thirteen

PEDIATRIC SURGERY

127

Pediatric (Infant) Laparotomy Set

ADD MINOR PLASTIC SET

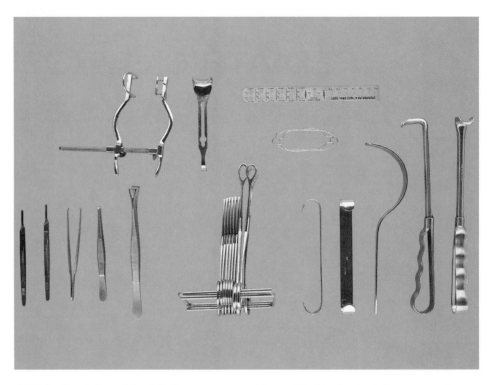

127-1 *Top, left to right,* 1 Balfour retractor with one bladder blade, infant; 1 metal ruler, 6 inch; 2 Spring retractors, 3 inch (hooked together, but used separately). *Bottom, left to right,* 2 Bard Parker knife handles, No. 9; 2 Cottle tissue forceps with teeth (4 × 5), front view, side view; 1 Wells tissue forceps, side view; 6 Allis tissue forceps, small; 2 Foerster sponge forceps, 7 inch; 2 Parker retractors, side view, front view; 1 Deaver retractor, extra small (infant); 2 Richardson retractors, small (infant).

Index